The Strength Code

by

Eric Falstrault

Dedication

My life and dedication to this way of life would have not been what they are today without the help of a few people. First and foremost, my parents, who thought me respect and punctuality, which have forged the basic principles of who I am today. They also never gave up on me, and they let me chose my calling.

Then came my friend and mentor Stephen, to whom I dedicate this work. He showed me more than any mentor could have shown me in a short but unforgettable friendship. We got separated by the often unstoppable disease that is cancer, but in the process he helped me become who I am today, a fearless and goal-driven individual. He showed me the way of the true warrior.

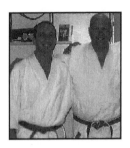

This is me and my sensei/mentor Steven Guy

Not to be forgotten is my strength mentor, Charles Poliquin. I have been following his advice for more than 15 years, and I can honestly say I wouldn't be as successful as I am today were it not for all his seminars, internships and courses that I attended throughout those years. I will always be grateful for everything I learned under his wing.

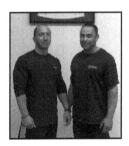

Picture or me and Charles Poliquin

And last but not least, my lovely wife, Cristina, and my beautiful kids, Matthew and Emily.

I know I have not been easy. I know I have worked a lot, daydreaming or stopping whatever I was doing, opening the computer and writing at any moment to avoid losing my train of thought. In fact, this is why I did this book, to help myself and others be better persons. I want to help and support the next generation by offering guidance and making sure they have a great foundation. Unfortunately, our generation will not make the future generation's life easier.

Chapter 1

The Lifestyle

Habits are what make or break you. It was always like that and always will be. However, changing habits takes guts and preparation, mentally and physically. It is a challenge in the first few days, or weeks, and it also challenges you physically at time due to hidden symptoms you didn't even know were related. This book will try to show you the why, the when, the what and the how of the challenging tasks of incorporating good habits back into your lifestyle and discarding the bad ones. On New Year's Day, it's always the same. People will make resolutions only to drop them a few weeks later. They make a dozen resolutions but fail to keep even one, and this is exactly where the problem lies.

Trying to change everything on the first day is doomed to failure from the get-go. What people fail to see is that habits are often fueled by other habits. For example, your goal is to quit eating your chocolate candies in the afternoon. Just trying to stop this habit may be easy in the short term, but to help you out, you may need to look at other things to understand WHY you need that little sugar boost in the afternoon.

After smoking, bedtime snacking is one of the most often sought habit changes for many people. Most people know it is one of the most damaging habits if you want to lose weight. But why is it so hard to stop? Willpower has a much to do with it, but what if you could do something to stop the hunger before going to bed? It's not as easy as it seems, but recognizing the symptoms that trigger these cravings can help you and can go a long way, not only by eliminating these bad habits but also in helping improve your health in the process.

I have found that changing a habit is almost like doing three sets of ten repetitions on the squat. The more you do, the more reps you try, the more weight you add. This kicks your ass every single time. The first set is fine, the second and third always get worse, or better in a sadistic sense. Changing habits is the same. The first time you try to lose weight for example, it's all good until you hit the wall. The second time, you know the wall is coming. This leaves you with two options: you try to break the wall, or you give up before you hit it. Most people give up before. Why? Trying to change habits is exhausting. So don't mistake laziness with exhaustion when the time comes to tackle new habits. It empties your self-control reserve since it depletes some automatic behaviors you had for years. When there is no more self-control, the mental muscles required to think creatively and focus on the task at hand are depleted. The more they persist, the more they tire out the mental muscles needed for new habits to kick in.

After talking with people and evaluating their needs for more than 20 years, I still can't put my finger on why it's so hard for people to put a foot down and take control of their lives. You must be able to trade your habits for healthier ones, get in shape, lift weights, work in a field you love instead of looking for security, all for the sake of money. Most people will settle for less just to make sure they get by and live with the minimum in terms of money. They are prepared to live a life that's less than ordinary just to live another day. Since you picked up this protocol and are more than ready to start, this leaves you ready for the next phase. The next few lessons, taken from ancient warriors, are in my opinion the epitome of a healthy and strong existence.

Warriors are warriors 24 hours a day, seven days a week. They follow the way of the samurai, bushido. This encompasses the concepts of sincerity, selflessness, cultural attainment, martial skills and the willingness to die for one's cause, which was made famous in the work of Hagakure. I stumbled onto a similar work from almost the same era as Hagakure. The difference was that instead of "not valuing one's own life" as the way of the warrior, the writer emphasized the warrior's strong body, mind and spirit. A samurai physician with philosophical and Buddhist learning, Kaibata Ekiken went the other way, taking the opposite approach. He understood that the physical, mental and spiritual aspects of great warriors were in fact all connected. He examined everything from nutrition to sexual practices, sustaining stamina from youth to old age, overindulgence and restraint, healthy habits, and much more.

The basic principle of Ekiken is that we are all born with a body meant to last 100 years. How we take care of it will determine whether we live to see our 100th birthday, live it to the fullest and enjoy it to the utmost. His ways of nurturing life were and still are highly respected, even after three centuries. I strongly suggest that you read his life work *Yojokun, Life lessons from a samurai*. Those life lessons are good not just for ancient samurai warriors. These are the habits that will forge a healthier and stronger body with all the resulting benefits in your daily life. Here are my top five lessons learned from Ekiken's way of nurturing life that could be applied nowadays to achieve a life worth living.

Lesson #1

Preserving life is a matter of what we eat. Food and drink are the nourishment of life. For this reason, nourishment should be considered a special daily supplement to one's life not to be neglected or abused. The stomach and spleen receive the nutrients that sends the pure liquid (pure liquid that supports animal life, that becomes blood) to the organs and viscera, just as the grass and trees grow due to the *ch'i* of the earth. In other words, taking care of the stomach is of the utmost importance in Yojokun (way of nurturing life) and in taking care of the body. The ancients always set limits to their food intake to avoid disrupting the balance, and this nourished their health. You must always be aware of what goes into your mouth. The ancients often said, "Disasters go out through the mouth and disease comes in through it." Food and drink should be used to extinguish hunger and thirst. Once this desire is fulfilled, you should stop eating. Control yourself and set limits.

Another great point is that you should write down all the things that consistently make you ill, and then avoid them. A consistent malady becomes a chronic illness. Some will make you ill immediately and others over time. Avoid both at all costs.

Lesson #2

Be grateful. Gratitude precludes envy and greed, cures anger, heals resentment, encourages a sense of contentment and promotes moderation, restraint and balance. Good health is what you owe to yourself but also to the world around you. Be grateful for your parents and nature itself that gives you all you need to sustain life. The highest ingratitude of all towards your parents and towards the society that educated and provided for you is to neglect your health.

Lesson #3

One of the first principles of Yojokun is to avoid overexposure to things that can damage your body. These may be divided into two categories, inner desires and external influences. Inner desires include food, drink, sex, sleep and excessive talking as well as the seven emotions, joy, anger, anxiety, yearning, sorrow, fear and astonishment. Negative external influences are the four dispositions of nature: wind, cold, heat and humidity. Being able to control your inner desires is the true foundation of the way of nurturing life. If you have a strong foundation, your strength will increase and you'll be able to hold off the external influences. However, lack of caution towards your desires will weaken your health and make you vulnerable to external influences that will most often result in serious illness and a shorter lifespan.

The essentials to nourish your mind and *ch'i* are:

- Suppress anger and desire.
- Diminish grief and yearning.
- Never trouble your mind nor your *ch'i*.
- Do not take excessive pleasure in sleep. *Ch'i* does not circulate well when lying down for extended periods of time.
- Never go to bed with a full stomach.
- Never eat until full, never go beyond moderation, and establish limits.
- Never sit, stand or lie down for a long time. Move to make the *ch'i* flow.

Lesson #4

There is an old saying that goes; "The sage treats the not-yet-ill," meaning that being careful beforehand will help avoid sickness altogether. Sun Tzu said, "The man who uses his army well performs no outstanding meritorious deeds." In other words, using your resources skillfully will avoid great and dangerous battles. He also stated that the ancients who were skillful at defeating the enemy were those who defeated the easily defeated. This is the way you should use Yojokun, committing yourself to being victorious (healthy) before the battle even begins (illness). This is the strategy to heal the not-yet-ill.

Lesson #5

One day at a time is the golden rule. Be circumspect of that day alone. Live and examine yourself one day at a time. By exhibiting common sense from morning to night, you will make no mistakes, cause little or no damage and suffer no disasters in your allotted span of life. Live for today: this will prepare your tomorrow.

Let's get out of the ancient mentality and get into our modern era.....

After a certain point in our lives, we need to prove ourselves. We need to get a reality check and start thinking about what if. What if we missed a hidden opportunity? What if we didn't choose the right path? To tell you the truth, I can say that I have beautiful kids, a wonderful wife, a house and a successful business, but why is it that this never seems enough? The fact is, I failed a number of times in various projects. I owned a private clinic where we had the chance to make it big, but we failed.

Although I don't like to blame others for our failures, it was justified in this instance. A bad partnership and a crooked investor led me towards failure. Was it something I didn't suspect? **I smelled problems from the get-go.** Why didn't I stop the problems before they started? Like most people, I thought, why not roll with the punches. Make the most of it, and see where this leads. They say we learn from our mistakes. I learned and still do. In fact, we all learn, and it's a never-ending work in progress.

After learning not only from myself but also from clients, I can say that, even though we control most of our lives, it's impossible to control 100% of our environment. There is always some kind of blockage, whether visible or not, immediate or not. Believing that we can control everything is insane. Believing that we can do everything possible to control our lives is possible. If you eat well, you can master your health. If you master your health, usually the mind follows. If the mind follows, then you can do almost anything. Your thoughts become clearer. What's funny is that you seem to interact differently with your surroundings, or they interact differently with you, which helps you control your environment and your surroundings.

The goal of this book is to share what I have learned from more than 15 years of coaching people from all walks of life. Showing them how to lead better lives, control their emotions and learn how to read their own hidden symptoms. This book will show you just that. Your body is yelling at you. If you can't hear what it has to say, you could lead a miserable life. You can master how you control your emotions, your surroundings, your health and your mind. I intend to give you the tools for you to use and to begin living the rest of your life the way you should.

In the following pages, you will see real-life everyday people, their major habits, their problems, the changes people want so badly, and everything you need to know to help you recognize the triggers and, I hope, to give you the tools to eradicate them completely from your life for good.

"When one is writing a letter, he should think that the recipient will make it into a hanging scroll."
— Yamamoto Tsunetomo, *Hagakure: The Book of the Samurai*

Chapter 2

Modern-Day Warriors

We all want proof. We learn from our mistakes and are motivated by success stories. Many warriors have followed these principles and have had these specific habits to live by. They swore by them and, if they failed to follow them or just went off track, they felt something was going to go terribly wrong. Think about a natural built-in obsessive-compulsive disorder. But this is not what it was. Let's take high-level athletes. They each have some sort of pre-game or pre-competition routine.

"Obsession is what lazy people call dedication."

That's exactly it. Some people call this an obsession, but it's what needs to be done for success. People know that, if their ritual is to have an afternoon nap, followed by a specific meal and listening to Metallica before jumping on the ice, if that sets the mood and fires them up for a great game, then why not? If you know that sleeping a seven-hour night will help you have a clear mind, why not do it? If your goal to lose ten pounds requires you to reserve your Sunday night in meal preparation instead of going out with friends, who may regard you as obsessed, why not do it? It's only until you have reached your goal. In my book, it's called dedication. So it's no secret that this code requires dedication and a fair amount of guts. Many who have been inspired by this code and who have switched to it have proven time and time again that anybody can do it. This includes people from all walks of life, not just warriors. This section will provide you with many real-life examples you can relate to. I think most of the valuable information in this book starts from their experiences, which arose from trial and error. As you will soon read, it was not an easy task.

> "Successful people are simply those with successful habits."
> — Brian Tracy

I have a tendency to remember most of my clients' and family members' symptoms. What I encounter the most is food intolerances. For the sake of clarification, there is a major difference between food intolerances and allergies. Allergies can trigger a severe reaction, which can often be fatal. However, intolerances will bring on mild symptoms or discomfort that can last and even appear only a few days later. In this case, it makes my job tougher and feeds my obsessive-compulsive disorder tendencies. Where am I going with this? As you will read later, repeating what I stated earlier, habits are fed by other habits. The trick is to recognize them and stop putting oil on the fire. Next is what I think many people can relate to, from the regular Joe to the elite Jock.

THE COACH

I've been doing this for a while now, and all I can say is that, thank God, I love what I do. Those who think that, once you get in shape, it only gets easier – these people are truly mistaken. We don't have the mind game of being halfway there, but a goal is still a goal. We all live through something called life. We get last-minute changes of plans, bad news and busier-than–expected schedules – all this seems to happen as we are trying to achieve a specific goal.

Six months ago, I decided to put my money into it. I booked a photo shoot with a professional team with what was supposed to be a few clients and friends. But as usual, most of those lazy bums changed their minds halfway through it. So I was left with one of my most serious clients, Robert, whom you will get to know later. As expected, our busiest time of the year had to arrive and mess with our goal.

Unfortunately, being crazy-busy was the least of my problems. Something pretty much messed up my cervical spine, with a major problem between C5, C6 and C7 from an old martial arts injury. So I had my work cut out for me. My biggest obstacle was the obvious pain in my neck, but I also lost a little over half the strength in my left elbow flexors and, as time went by, it started affecting my left tricep as well. I was not a happy camper, at all.

I saw all kinds of specialists, but I knew that only my buddy osteopath could fix me up. I remembered that once, he told me that I had to work on my diaphragm (which I obviously failed to do). All I wanted and felt like I needed was a good crack in the cervical area and the problem would be fixed. It turned out I was right, but not without a complicated way through it. The problem started at the sigmoid, which inhibited the proper functioning and movement of my first thoracic rib (don't ask me why, that's why I refer to him). Once that was taken care of, mobility was better and we finally could crack that mother bumper, which was impossible to do before. Believe me when I say we tried it before (with no shortage of pain). When it cracked, it felt like a river started flowing back down my arm and zapping my fingers. I immediately felt everything coming back. But the strength wasn't there, and I had to work my way up to normal slowly. For example, I was not even able to do a 45-degree Scott curl with a 15-pound dumbbell six months ago with my left arm. (Now I am back up to 55 pounds for reps.)

All that, happened in the first three months. Then things got better, and I saw results slowly every week, which was my initial intent, not rushing into it but going with the flow. My ultimate goals were (and still are) to stay in top shape, year round, without all the nonsense spewed in blogs, on Facebook or wherever some fitness freaks may turn.

I truly don't give a crap about what so-called specialists say or what study they shove in my face. Eat nutrient-dense foods, get stronger, move, live, enjoy a great and happy life, and make time for people you love and for your passions. That, in my opinion, is living a healthy, strong and awesome life.

The thing is that, for the past few years, I have been following this code. Studying, learning, gathering information from everyone's consultations and habits, understanding them as best I can – this is the way I learned how I, or we, can have some sort of control over what we do and how we think every day. Almost everyone can do it to. I say "almost" because it does not happen overnight. You must learn, apply and repeat. I have studied old-time warriors, along with the new breed. I have practiced among them, learned from them and got into their heads.

All that we do has an impact on our quality of life, like a chain and its entire links. Everything is connected. If we break a link, the rest becomes fragile, the chain becomes weaker and the load is shifted onto every other link.

As you will soon find out, the greatest and most successful warriors / samurai / coaches / executives / entrepreneurs have been following those very same habits and way of life in order to achieve greatness in their everyday lives, which became worth living. It may have taken them a while to figure out the code, how to deal with it and, ultimately, how to live by it. I follow it and it is now available for everyone seeking to achieve their goals and enjoy the best of health for as long as they can hold onto "the strength code."

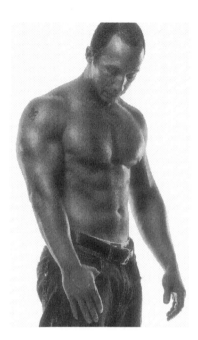

THE LAWYER

I've been training a friend of mine on and off for the last 15 years. She was there when I started working in gyms, and she is still there now. I watched her study her head off to get into law school, and she became very successful at it. Her shape at that time was okay, but nothing sensational, and she felt it. She was a cardio fanatic. She regularly went on the elliptical for 30 to 45 minutes, talking with her cardio female companions, four to five times a week. Let me remind you that this was some 15 years ago. I didn't know as much as I do now, but I knew that weightlifting was a much better alternative to doing cardio. She has always been changing her programs every month or so, and my job was to keep her motivated. She went to see other trainers, but she always came back to me.

Let's fast-forward to the last two years. She always retained fat, mainly in the lower body, with a lean and even cut upper body when she is able to stick to the plan. She took contraceptive pills for many years, but she knew and felt that this was becoming a problem in her fat loss results. I showed her from month to month how it affected her, physically and mentally. She had the highest of highs (mentally and physically) for two weeks, and then she fell as low as she could mentally for the other two weeks. She couldn't put her thoughts together, and I constantly had to remind her when she felt like shit and when she felt good. It's a good thing I remember almost every symptoms and brain fart of all my clients. Some days she came in and took charge. Other days, she was almost crying with dismal motivation and attitude. The problem with the pill is that it can elevate estrogen or cause an imbalance between estrogen and other hormones.

This caused her to blame everybody and everything, and sometimes, herself. The problem lay in the "sometimes." Blaming everyone and every situation is what most people do, and in her case the problem was also her surroundings. You are whom you hang around the most with. You may find yourself hanging around people who tell you:

- *Eating meat is no good for you; you'll die of cancer.*
- *You should do more cardio; you look like you gained mass.*
- *Doing no cardio at all can't be good for you; how can you lose weight then?*
- *I love Weight Watchers; I can eat what I want, as long as I don't eat fat.*

Now, once she got below 12% and got the shape she always wanted.

- *Are you sure that's good for you? You've lost a lot of weight.*
- *I don't like meat; I don't understand how you do it.*
- *Are you sure eating all that fat is good for you?*

By the way, does this sound familiar?

Even though she is always training hard, some days I would slap her behind the head - with a Mack truck - twice. Because of her friends who forced her to drink, not intentionally, no sirree bob. Just because social drinking is what it is. If you don't drink, others will give you a weird look, suggesting you are no fun, etc. It's also her fault: nothing goes into your mouth by accident.

One day, something clicked. She decided to take charge, stopped the pill and started her "new life." Did I believe her? Hell no! Now let's go to the last year or so. In one of those bad weeks, and one of my "don't piss on my shoes and tell me it's raining" morning mood, I got fed up. I told her to put up or shut up, that I was done with her and that I didn't want to see her again in my gym. This is one of the downsides of training friends. You tell them to fuck off, and it only means to get out of my face. Then everything is fine the next day. But this time, I was serious. She fought back with every excuse, and I didn't see her for two weeks.

I took her back after that. She trained more than she ever did on her own in those two weeks, and something changed. Since that time, she bumped up her training to four or five times a week, with amazing dedication. I still give her a hard time, but she does what is expected. She listens to common sense. Not that she didn't know anything before. I teach and preach as best I can to every single client I have, but now, she found a way to answer back, to prove her shit. She is now in the best shape of her life and maintains her body fat at about 10% year round.

Not bad for someone who thought that 20% body fat was what life gave her and that she couldn't change a thing about it. What she did is change her attitude. She learned to understand how her body works and finally learned to listen to her body. Loss of energy, sleep disturbance and every little symptom can say a lot on what your body goes through. She also does what I do most of the time, selective hearing. Take in the good information and discard what makes no sense. How does she know what's good or not? Experience! Nothing beats that. I showed her everything she NEEDED to know, and threw away what she WANTED to hear. Results are the best way to prove a point. Nothing but hard work can bring you to them. She is one of my proudest achievements.

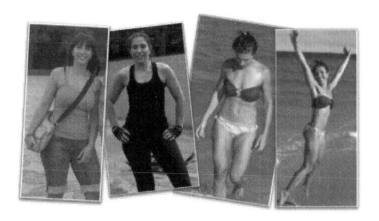

THE SUPERMOM

Another real-life example I can give you is a new client I just started working with. Niki never lost weight, even if she wanted to. She has tried everything (didn't everybody?), and not even doctors can figure out what is wrong with her. Doctors are good for one thing, to help you once you are sick. My job is the step before. I have to work on prevention. Make sure you don't get to the point of needing a doctor, ever. Doctors will never be obsolete; they just fail to let people know the basics. Not because they don't want to: it's just that they don't have enough time. All she kept saying was that she couldn't bring her weight lower than 260 pounds. After four weeks, she lost six pounds to bring her to 254. So the psychological barrier has been broken. The first major habit I tried to break is regular scale "humping." Every single morning, most people will get on the scale and weigh themselves. The fact of the matter is that your weight will fluctuate a lot throughout the week. For those who are weight-sensitive, meaning that they eat according to what they weigh, it will play with their head and can only lead to an unhealthy relationship with food.

As I started training her frequently, I began to discover who she was. The everyday superhuman mom. Helped her husband with a successful business, playing taxi with her daughter, juggling between gym and home, taking care of her parents and business and trying to find time to eat on the corner of the table, when she found the time, that is. Once we started training, she still had some major headaches, the same she has had for years. The problem was that they were becoming worse and worse. As with any new trainee, I start by incorporating a few lifestyle changes. In her case, one of them was eating a better breakfast. Most of the time, she skipped breakfast, and when she eats in the morning, she had a piece of toast or a fat-free yogurt. After the second week, something was up. It turned out she had been eating eggs every single morning, which was feeding her eggs intolerance. How did we figure out she had an intolerance to eggs? We just let them go, and her headaches have been gone since the last time she ate them. Her weight is now going down slowly. She is starting to feel a lot better, and also, sees a difference in her clothes and daily energy levels.

THE TRAINER WHO GOT TRAINED

Here's a cardio-cereals-marathon-organic-thought-she-was-in-shape client of mine who completely changed her shape and career and turned around everything having to do with what she loves. She is a great trainer on her way up to a great coaching career. Who better than she herself to explain what she first experienced in an experienced trainer's office?

"Where do I begin? It was about three years ago when I first stepped into Eric's office. At the time, I was a spinning instructor for the same gym and worked for an investment firm. (I have a university degree in finance.) Today, I'm still a spinning instructor, and I have left the world of finance to do what I am truly passionate about, helping people attain optimal health. This is relevant because it explains how I met Eric and why I chose to become a personal trainer as well.

After a couple of years teaching four spinning classes a week, training for two half-marathons and a full marathon (I never made it to attend the full marathon, and looking back now, thank God I didn't), weight training once or twice a week, and whatever other physical activity I engaged my body in, I had started to feel the "symptoms" of what many would assume to be some sort imbalance in my body. Although it was never clear to me at first, maybe because I was in denial, or maybe because I was convinced I wasn't exercising too much and that I was eating properly, or maybe because I'm hard-headed and often think I know everything. The symptoms were clearly apparent, but not to me. In fact, even the loss of my menses weren't enough to convince me that my body was in a state of hormonal havoc. Weird how the mind works sometimes!!

Anyhow, for all these reasons and more, I was caught in a vicious circle. Like any other women on this earth, I wasn't satisfied with my body; I wanted to get leaner. So I was constantly obsessing about eating and exercising, reading every book I could possibly find on nutrition (obviously the wrong ones, most of the time by registered dieticians or nutritionists, or even MDs). Basically, I figured I could train as much as I wanted, as long as I ate accordingly, and that it was healthy (whatever that meant at the time). And so I went on and trained (cardio) excessively. The more I trained, the hungrier I was and the more I ate. The more I ate, the hungrier I was getting... And still no period. I thought to myself, if I'm eating so much, why would I still not get my period.

To make sense of it all, I need to clarify what my so called "healthy diet" consisted of: the all-so-famous ORGANIC cereals (apparently, because they are organic they are good for us), whole wheat toast, egg whites, low-fat yogurt (even low-fat Greek yogurt), skim milk, low-fat cheese (Yuk! Low-fat cheese doesn't even sound appetizing), some nuts, a bit of olive oil, chicken breast, turkey breast, fish, red meat (no more than twice a month, because my doctor had told me it wasn't good for me), and that's about it. In all, my diet consisted of about 50% to 60% carbs, 30% to 35% protein, and a very low percentage of fat (specifically saturated and monounsaturated fats).

I was confused. I visited many doctors and did numerous blood tests and ultrasounds, but no one could figure out what was going on. Doctors' solutions: eat more, train less, get on the pill and so on. Oh, and I forgot, "gain weight, your body fat is too low." I was 122 pounds and I'm 5'2". I'm not skinny. I must have been around 19% to 20% body fat. And to top it off, one doctor actually thought I was anorexic. Anyway, through a coworker, I was told to go see Eric. And so I did.

I'm not sure I should share with you what my first impressions of Eric were. Although at first they might appear to go against the point of a testimonial, keep reading. I assure you there is a point to all this writing.

Let just say that, for that hour when we met for the first time, he told me to eliminate cereals (even the ORGANIC ones), breads (even whole wheat), starches (including grains — all gluten-containing products), milk and dairy products (even the low-fat ones), legumes, soy products and instead to add more lean red meats and fats (butter, coconut oil, avocados) to whatever protein I was already consuming. For the entire duration of our first meeting, I kept repeating in my head: "This guy has to be kidding. He just ripped me off, AND he's wasting my time trying to convince me that doctors, nutritionists, dietitians and even the Canadian Food Guide have it all wrong. He's an idiot. And he probably thinks I'm an idiot." Anyhow, I figured, since I had paid the guy, I'd train with him anyways and we'll see what happens. And obviously, close to no results. I didn't trust him!! I couldn't commit to his BioSignature program. How could I follow his guidelines if I didn't think it would work??

I'll be honest, I thought he was an arrogant guy, who was so convinced that he knew it all and that his approach was the only way to go and that if you didn't believe in what he believed in, well than, you were worthless! So I didn't trust him, I couldn't trust what he was preaching. How could it make sense, if all of these professionals with recognized diplomas followed different guidelines I couldn't believe him, and his attitude turned me off. He was too narrow-minded for me. So, I couldn't commit to his diet, to his training. I didn't trust his knowledge. SO I stuck with my hard head and did my own thing.

This is why it failed, because I failed to trust him.

I eventually went out on my own again, started reading the right books. After two years of trial and error, I finally found a way of eating that is the exact replica of what Eric preaches. I toned it down on the cardio (something Eric must have repeated to me too many times for me to have kept count) and replaced it with something else I am also passionate about, yoga (I am a certified Hatha Yoga instructor). And I finally got my period. No wonder this arrogant prick was so narrow-minded and believed so much in what he was doing. After all, who wouldn't? If you know that what you dedicate your life to actually does help improve people's health and their lives, why wouldn't you be so narrow-minded?

So, I changed my diet, relaxed on the cardio, integrated yoga in my everyday life and Eric now trains me three times a week. Having left the finance field to dedicate my time to what I love to do, I must confess that I couldn't have chosen a better mentor then Eric. Every day I learn something new with him. He lives for what he does.

Thank you Eric and keep up the great work. Your efforts and sacrifices are mirrored on every single client of yours."
Tania

THE YOUNG AND THE RESTLESS

Believe it or not, this is the toughest crowd. They know it all, everything you tell them has to be cool but, thank God, they see results fast. Young ones fortunately don't have habits. They are still in discovery mode and, as soon as it sounds like a routine or habit, they seem to change it very fast instinctively. Getting them at the right time is the key.

Enter the teen figure skating world for a minute and all the healthy notions takes a hike. Their coaches are so far behind with their nutritional knowledge that I would rather follow the advice of Barney than to listen to them. Many problems seem to be the same as the runway model world: all they think about is losing weight. Teaching the parent, the coach and then the kid is very interesting since, if one of them don't get in the game, nothing will ever get done. Even though it doesn't look like it, the sport requires a great deal of strength and plenty of discipline and focus. The high forces on the knee joints requires the best nutrient support possible through a great nutrition plan and an individualized training program which, in the figure skating world, is somewhat rare. You can't take five girls, make them do the same plan (nutrition and/or training) and expect the same results from all five of them. Training them and treating them as individuals is of the utmost importance. You need to focus on your own difficulties without comparing yourself to anyone else. That was the first habit change that I needed to apply. Making them eat more than a butterfly was the next big change to apply.

Girls will be girls. The way they look is more important then how they feel, and I won't even talk about peer pressure or, more often than I care to see, parental pressure. I have to make sure that they have the proper psychological support before starting to incorporate nutritional changes or, as I said, it won't work. Once the kid and the parent understand the importance of optimal nutrient support in their plan, half the job is done, and the rest is in their hands. These habits or changes are somewhat different from what you'll see in the remaining examples, but in my book, different individuals always equal different needs.

THE PROFESSIONAL

Robert has two careers or, I should say, one working job and a passion. I have known him for many years, and his drive for anything or project he undertakes is constant, and he never gives up. He is a mortgage specialist in a very well known bank, and he has won the title of best seller in North America on multiple occasions. His passion is dancing. He is partner with Marie-Josée Strazzero, an internationally known dancer. This makes him a mortgage specialist by day and a professional dancer and teacher by night. He always came to me in preparation for a big show or just to put him back in good shape. In his case, my problem was that he is Italian. Meh! What's a matter you? You talkin' to me? All the clichés about Italian, as to how they exaggerate with food and baking stuff is often true.

If you are too skinny, the Nonnas want you to gain weight and will practically feed you until you burst. If you are fat and stuffed, you are healthy and big-boned. If you don't eat their food, they will be offended, so never mess with the Nonnas. Have you ever watched The Sopranos? Foget about it. I gained and bought all the rights to make fun and take a poke at them because I married an Italian woman, so I clearly know what I am talking about. This also helped me understand Robert's background and how to deal with it.

Like most people, Robert thought he ate well. The problem is that my definition of eating well is really different from how others see it. Some think that eating fruit and a piece of bagel in the morning is eating well. A bowl of organic kashi, which in fact are full of GMOs, can make your muffin top even worse. In Robert's case, the problem lay in lack of the right nutrients. Most professionals and executives think toast and coffee in the morning is enough for them to function or that Wheaties breakfast cereal is the actual breakfast of champions. Nothing could be further from the truth. Robert was the "toast if I have time" kind of guy. If you looked at the rest of the day, he was eating well, with the usual salads and some kind of meat (whatever was alive before) at lunch and dinner. The problem was the caloric deficit. I don't believe in the calories in = calories out notion, but sometimes a balance needs to be found. You can't expect your body to function properly when you train like a horse but eat like a bird. Robert is working full time, teaches dancing for three hours almost every night and is also dancing and practicing for himself for upcoming competitions and shows. Add this to the multiple weightlifting sessions we do in a week, and there's a whole lot of moving going on.

Here are some of the little adjustments I did to his lifestyle. One of the first habits I change with people is their breakfast. The first thing you eat dictates how your body will function for the rest of the day. Once I proved to him that toast and coffee was not the breakfast of choice, I started changing his definition of eating well. The followings are some of Robert's and also, most people's, definition of eating well.

- Salads are good enough (for rabbits). Lettuce or any kind of leafy salads are great, but unfortunately not enough for most of us. Add some green veggies such as broccoli, cauliflower, or any big vegetables. Much better for your health and digestive system.

- Three meals a day is good enough (for a 12-year-old ballerina). We have to feed our body according to the amount of activity we get. About 80% of the population eats maybe two big meals a day, with the major one at night, when they sit on their ass and start contemplating bed. Four equally balanced meals spread throughout the day will help the body use energy wisely and, believe it or not, burn fat. Sumo wrestlers eat two huge meals a day and sleep after each one of them. Would you want to look like them? It's funny how most people don't want to look like sumo wrestlers but actually eat like them.

- Breads and pasta: Italians have a special relationship with these foods. As a matter of fact, most people do. Breads and baked products are a staple in the average American diet, which is, in my opinion, the culprit of today's obesity pandemic. To put it simply, if you bake it and it rises like bread and cakes in the oven, it does the same exact thing with your belly. It disturbs your digestive system in many ways and actually can make you intolerant to many foods, good or not. Gluten has got a lot of bad rap these years, and it's only going to get worst. Only about 10% of the population can tolerate gluten, and the only true test for knowing if you are intolerant is to avoid it for at least three weeks. What food does contain gluten? It is easier for me to enumerate what does not. Eat organic meats, veggies and healthy fats at each meal for three weeks. If you feel better, see your stomach go down and energy level improve, you found the answer. The last part of the test is to try to eat some bread. If you feel like shit after and see an almost immediate response in your energy level, and if your stomach inflates like a balloon, then, my friend, you are intolerant.

These small but very important changes improved Robert's health tremendously. With his busy schedule, we were only able to fit in three weightlifting sessions a week. At first we started to lift weights in a circuit style to make him burn fat. He was running about two days a week, and I actually make him stop for a while, as it was getting him nowhere (pun intended). Contrary to popular belief, running is not the best choice if you want to lose FAT! Yes, you burn calories, but weightlifting is a better long-term tool. By gaining lean muscle mass, you increase your metabolism. If you increase your metabolic rate, you increase your chances of burning fat. Considering running uses up a lot of energy and that most people don't eat even close to the amount of calories they should when they practice running as a physical activity, they lose muscle mass, which turns out to be counterproductive if you want to lose fat, for good. Here is a vivid example: which shape would you rather have, a sprinter or a long-distance runner?

His training was like what I would give to a bodybuilder, training three body parts a day split as follows:

Chest / back / shoulders
Quadriceps / hamstrings / calves
Biceps / triceps / forearms

As soon as you mention the word bodybuilding, most people react the same way they think they will gain muscle mass as fast as any champion bodybuilder on the planet. As if they have some kind of special superhero ability to pump muscles up like crazy just by lifting weights. The same goes for girls to whom I often give this kind of program. Most girls want to look like a fitness model but don't want to train like one. The thing with this type of training is that it's easy on the nervous system and, as I mentioned earlier, it helps boost your metabolism.

Even though people think that as soon as they lift weights they gain lean mass, gaining ten pounds of lean muscle won't really show on a person's frame, unlike ten pounds of fat, which actually stores in specific places like the butt and stomach. Gains in muscle will always result in a better shape and some type improved muscle quality and definition. Often people don't lose weight at all on the scale but their shape changes drastically. They could have gained ten pounds of muscle but lost the same amount of fat, resulting in zero difference on the scale but improved health and overall shape. So in Robert's case, it helped him in many ways. It improved almost every aspect of his life. It was easier to lift his dancing partners, and it improved his stamina while dancing. Remember, this was the same guy who used to run once or twice a week for cardio purposes. He maintains a healthy body fat percentage year round and can still manage to be the best at what he does for a living.

THE ELITE

Elite athlete, that is. One of my elite clients is the best goalie in the National Hockey League, Martin Brodeur, No. 30 with the New Jersey Devils. In case you are not a fan, here is a little bit of what he accomplished.

In 20 seasons, he has set NHL records for most games played by a goalie (1,220), most wins (669), most shutouts (121), most saves made (30,569) and most minutes played (71,786). He has the most 30-win (14) and 40-win (eight) seasons in league history.

Along the way he's won the Stanley Cup three times. He has also captured four Vezina trophies, five Jennings trophies, two Olympic gold medals and a World Cup of Hockey championship.

Brodeur played more than 70 games in a season for ten straight seasons, from 1997 to 2008, but in 2008-09 he sustained his first major injury, tearing the biceps tendon in his left elbow, which sidelined him four months.

He came back and helped the Devils get into the playoffs. The following season, at age 37, he led the League in games played (77), wins (45), and shutouts (nine), and was third with a 2.24 goals-against average.

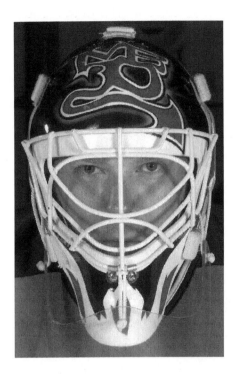

I started working with him the year before, in the 2007-08 season. The big injury was devastating news, since he entered the season in perfect game shape. However, true soldier that he is, he kept on with the plan, and recovered in half the time this type of injury usually takes, thanks to proper nutrients and the optimal supplement protocol.

We started working together after one of my friends introduced Brodeur to some of my work. Marty, although not out of shape after many years of being an NHL goaltender, felt he needed to improve some aspects of his off-season preparation. As he was getting older, he felt it was getting a bit harder to get fit enough for training camp. That is when I came into the picture. The first time he came to my office, the guy looked every inch an elite athlete should be, tall, imposing and fit. My guess was that it wasn't going to be hard to show him a few tricks and get him in even better shape. Those guys are machines of habits. If you ever had the chance to talk to them, you see very fast that they have a routine and that their habits can change much of their mindset. So for that reason, I had to be very specific and clear about what and why I had to change some of his habits.

He's been at the top of the game for many years. This speaks volumes as to what he has been doing throughout those years to stay at that level. Although I was speaking with the best there is, my approach didn't change. I asked the same questions I would with a regular Joe. My biggest mistake would have been to skip the basics and assume that he was fine. First and foremost, everyone I take on has to pass an evaluation, physical as well as nutritional.

For instance, one of the tools I use is the Poliquin bio-signature concept. As we take body fat readings, we know by order of priority which hormones to manipulate in order to maximize the body's ability to lose fat and gain muscle mass optimally, with nutrition and supplements if needed. During that evaluation, one of the first things I look at is breakfast. Most athletes think that eating oatmeal or yogurt in the morning is great, but I disagree. Sure, it's a better choice than eating Nutella spread but, depending on goals, I may have to advise otherwise. When I have to lower someone's body fat, I initially take out most carbohydrates, such as refined sugar, grains and cereals, in other words, all man-made foods. First thing in the morning come protein and fat. As the day advances, the body has an easier time breaking down carbohydrates. However, the goals determine the process. In his case, we needed to lose body fat so I had to cut down on simple carbohydrates, especially those needing plenty of insulin to break down, such as oatmeal. The problem with oatmeal is the cross-contamination of gluten. Since it is always transported with oats and wheat, there is always trace of gluten in oatmeal, unless specified otherwise.

Next was his pre-game meal ritual. Like most hockey players, eating carbs before a game is some kind of ritual. So the plate of pasta is like a religion for most of them. The problem with this is the sudden energy crash after a couple of minutes or hours later. Adding protein to this meal slows down the high insulin secretion it usually requires, and it suddenly delivers a steady and sustainable amount of energy that lasts a few hours, which makes it the ideal pre-game meal. For even better results, changing white flour pasta to gluten-free pasta was also a better alternative for him. However, since they are on the road more often than not, he does his best to take in the best meal for constant energy during the game.

The off-season is a whole other story. I have ten to 12 weeks to prepare him before training camp, all-out training four days a week with golf games every day and full nutritional boot camp limiting carbs to about 100 grams a day. His training sessions look nothing like his in-season maintenance protocol. I split the summer into 4 phases, which lasts about 3 to 4 weeks each, depending on how much time I have with them.

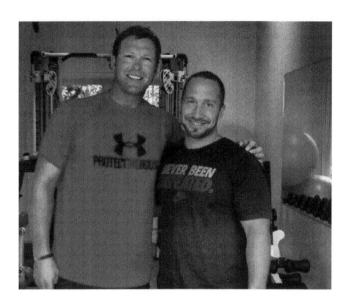

The first phase is where we focus on diet and structural balance. The initial evaluation is where all goals are set for the offseason and determines what work needs to be done structurally for a safe offseason and to reach our goals.

The second phase is most often used for lean muscle mass gain or fat loss. Even if this phase has already been started in phase one, this phase will focus more on individual goals, such as a player who would have lost a lot of lean mass during the season due to the constant travelling, the goal would be to gain back his lean muscle tissue.

The third phase is for strength. This phase prioritize the basic lifts such as Olympic lifts, squats, benchpress and pull-ups/chin ups. Olympic lifts are in my opinion a must when it comes to hockey preparation due the high recruitment of the posterior chain and its high efficiency to improve strength and power. I also incorporate strongman type trainings for the overall functional aspect of it, and I am not talking about instability training such as the swiss ball or bosu, which unfortunately has been wrongfully tagged as functional training tools. The body's ability to utilize a chain of muscle groups to develop maximum strength and power, which is the definition of functional training.

The fourth and last phase is strictly for power. The more powerful the athlete, the faster he will be on the ice. On top of being more powerful, it puts them in the right frame of mind to attack the pre camp and the approaching regular season.

Off-season is designed to fix up injuries, if any, and to prepare for the upcoming training camp in early September. Thankfully, he keeps his body fat at a 10% to 12% average year round. Whatever he learned from me, he applies year round.

The convictions

I have nothing against special diets or lifestyles and I truly believe that everyone can find their special way to help them achieve their goals. However, if you undertake a certain lifestyle and it is not giving you results or better health, don't waste your time. This next little tale is a true story.

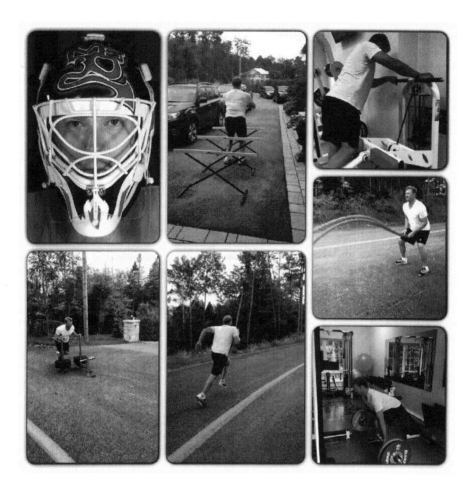

Nicole is a friend of mine and became a vegetarian because of a YouTube video she saw on how they treat animals in mass production meat factories. When she told me, I understood her concern and decided to respect her decision on becoming a vegetarian. Even though I don't agree with this way of life, I told her some of the downfalls of adopting such a lifestyle, like a lack of essential nutrients and possible health concerns. She went on and, for many years, followed this lifestyle. Goals remain the same, anyway, and she had to respect the guidelines. As the years went by, I saw her health deteriorating. Substantial loss of muscle mass is usually a good sign of problems to come. Was it a lack of protein? Nutrients? It was both and much more. The problem with those who adopt this lifestyle is that, even though they know for a fact that their health is showing some signs of decline, they persuade themselves that this is okay, sometimes saying something as stupid as, "Well at least, I don't make animals suffer" just to show that they are true soldiers. Dead soldiers are worthless soldiers in my book.

This is how I saw her health decline. She looked worse and worse. Her skin was yellowish, she had frequent anxiety attacks, her job performance was declining, with constant brain fog, and her body composition was getting nowhere. She was also having some concerns about her hormonal system as she was getting early menopausal symptoms, at age 28. She tried to train as best she could, but her energy levels were in the minuses.

That is when I gave her two options: change her lifestyle or find another trainer. Drastic, but I warned her from Day One that she might have some health problems adopting this kind of diet. I will not work with someone whose lifestyle interferes with my advice and results. After a few weeks of pouting, she came back and followed some of my suggestions.

If for humanitarian or animal cruelty reasons you choose not to eat meat, you can also rely on organic farms that treat their animals as in the olden days. All animals are free-range and hormone-free. Once she started eating protein, she IMMEDIATELY felt different. In a matter of days, she told me that her head and thoughts were clearer. She craved meat as soon as she finished her first solid protein meal. It has been almost a year now that she has been eating organic meats, and she is feeling much stronger, with energy levels skyrocketing, and she is as beautiful as can be. Her training sessions are way tougher than what I used to give her. Everything is back to normal again, and her body fat is below the 10% mark year round. She is no athlete, but she just takes her health and well being seriously.

Unfortunately, we are the top of the food chain, and it has always been like that. For thousands of years we relied on protein to survive. It's a fact that we can live a long time without carbs, but only a few weeks without protein.

Although I believe that animal protein is essential, I have came across individuals who adopted the vegetarian life and had amazing results with no signs of concern. As I said earlier, different individuals equals different needs. I personally am a vegetarian; I simply choose to eat animal protein with my tons of veggies.

Chapter 3

The Blueprint

Clear goals for success

In order to induce change, the right mindset needs to be set up. Following the lifestyle lessons enumerated previously will greatly help you get into fighting mode. However, the need for clear goals is fundamental before any type of change gets going.

For example, when someone tells me he wants to lose weight, the first thing that comes up to mind is whether he can be any more vague. The exact same thing goes for trainers. If the first question you ask someone is as vague as "Do you eat well?" chances are you'll get a vague answer. No wonder why some clients are resistant to change. Resistance often reflects a lack of clarity.

Keep the fire alive

To illustrate my point on self-control depletion, psychologist Roy Baumeister reflects on his 1998 research on self-control. Together with Ellen Bratslavsky, Mark Muraven, and Dianne Tice, his former Case Western Reserve University colleagues, he examined the effect of a tempting food challenge designed to deplete participants' willpower through the awful power of an unfulfilled promise of chocolate. How cruel!

In the first part of the trial, Baumeister kept the 67 study participants in a room that smelled of freshly baked chocolate cookies and then teased them further by showing them the actual treats alongside other chocolate-flavored confections. While some did get to indulge their sweet tooth, the subjects in the experimental condition, whose resolves were being tested, were asked to eat radishes instead. Many of the radish-eaters had a really hard time resisting the temptation to eat the chocolates. Some even picked up pieces of chocolate to sniff at them.

After the food bait-and-switch, Baumeister's team gave the participants a second and supposedly unrelated exercise, unsolvable puzzles. The effect of the manipulation was immediate and undeniable. Those who ate radishes made far fewer attempts and devoted less than half the time solving the puzzle compared to the chocolate-eating participants and a control group that only joined this latter phase of the study. In other words, those who had to resist the sweets and force themselves to eat pungent vegetables could no longer find the will to engage fully in another torturous task. They were already too tired.

Your next logical question should be: "How do we fill up our reserves? How do we get back our willpower and make sure we don't dig in those reserves?" What we do every day has an impact, and we must feed whatever needs to be fed, emotionally, physically or intellectually, to satisfy our lack of willpower. We require homeostasis to function optimally. Achieving it can be tricky and at times, almost impossible, but keeping close to it is not. All we need is to shape the path.

Let's shape the path...

What will follow is what I, and many other strength coaches around the planet, aim for, not only changing people's life in the short term, but primarily for the rest of their lives. We all have goals. However, the road to these goals will be full of trials and tribulations. The least we can do is to aim along the way to control every other element. When we set our sight on a specific and clear goal, a plan needs to be written and organized. In my technical and practical training as a close protection agent, a simple trip from Point A to Point B could be a plan from hell, depending on where we were. Every single detail had to be considered. For Plan A, we had a Plan 1, 2 and 3 for every possible situation we could imagine and prevent. The same goes for Plan B and the connected Plans B-1, B-2 and B-3. Reaching your goal doesn't have to be all that complicated, but I'm sure you understand where I am going with this.

The more elements you can control outside the simple fact of reaching your goal, namely being as strong and healthy as one can be, the better your chances are of reaching your goal faster and staying in that state, the alpha state, as long as you would like.

The main goal of the protocol is to change one's lifestyle, slowly, one step at a time. Unlike most people with their New Year's resolutions, they try to change too many habits all at once, which is the main reason most people fail in the first few weeks.

This protocol can be converted into a 12-week plan, or it can be converted into a longer plan such as a 12-month plan. The 12 habits will be the foundation of the protocol. They will be the ultimate goal. The plan is to change bad habits you may have, one week at a time. What you will need to do is find a goal that can be done in 12 weeks. Whether it is to lose 10-15 pounds or to gain ten pounds of muscle by changing most of your habits to support your daily workouts paired with your nutritional plan to reach your ultimate goal, you will find that your training sessions will be better, your diet easier and results will show up steadily and constantly.

Let's start with:

Habit #1: A healthier breakfast

Although this is unconventional, I would strongly suggest the Poliquin meat and nuts Breakfast™. Charles Poliquin himself introduced me to this concept many years ago. The most important habit to change is to eat properly and wisely in the morning. However, don't get caught up with what you think is good for you. Most people think that eating a bowl of cornflakes or Special K can help them get their sources of fibers and help lower their cholesterol. The insulin spike from cereals and grains is not worth the effort, especially in the morning. It will put you through a series of ups and downs throughout the day that promotes your fat-storing abilities.

People who changed their breakfast with the meat and nuts breakfast are the ones who got the most results, in both the short and long term. Why? They give their body a fighting chance by starting the day with the right kind of nutrients. My favorite is some type of red meat such as bison, grass-fed beef or any type of wild game with a serving of nuts. The first portion of protein of the day goes towards detoxification process, and it boosts your metabolism and immune system. If you ask me how much, I will tell you to eat as much as you can eat without feeling full. Don't be stressed about the amount. Start by eating what you can and work your way up from there.

If you someone who skips breakfast, you just make things worst. Even though research tends to show contradicting evidence, It was proven that those who skip breakfast eat more calories through-out the day. The logic is pretty simple to understand: since you lack a significant amount of calories, your body will send you sig-nals to compensate and to put some aside, leading to uncontrollable cravings.

The best way to burn fat and make sure you burn fat efficiently after your workout is to eat a good nutrient-dense breakfast before working out. A recent study from Italy found that training on an empty stomach is less efficient than eating a light meal consisting of protein and healthy fats. Researchers compared the effect of having young men run for 38 minutes at a moderate intensity of 65% of maximum heart rate after eating breakfast or skipping it.

The breakfast group lost 14% more fat than the group that fasted. Results showed that the group that ate breakfast burned significantly more fat for fuel during the workout (14% more). Fat oxidation was ideal during the 24-hour recovery period following the workout as well, meaning they continued burning fat, throughout the 24 hours after the workout. They concluded that eating breakfast prior the workout will enhance the fat-burning process.

When it comes to meat eating, the only thing you should be very meticulous about is the quality of the protein. Wild game or grass-fed beef are the best choices, even the ever-so-reliable eggs. However, I found that more and more people have some kind of intolerance to eggs: avoid overeating them. I suggest that you rotate your proteins and nuts. Never eat the same breakfast for more than two days. There are so many advantages to starting your day with such a breakfast that, in the end, you'll ask yourself why you didn't start earlier. One of the benefits is that the L-Carnitine in the meat and the tyrosine and good fats from the nuts will boost brain capacity and concentration. You don't believe me? Give it a fair try for a couple of days. You'll feel a difference and maybe see one in your mid-section as well.

I know it's hard to change your habits, especially that one, but I am convinced that this particular habit is one that can and that will improve your day like nothing else. I truly believe that most people are gaining weight just because they don't start the day with the proper nutrients. Here's some additional info about the meat and nuts breakfast and the Paleolithic lifestyle.

Cause and effect: Those who have a hard time having breakfast or just being hungry in the morning are usually the late-night snack nibblers. Unless you have very fast metabolism, snacks just before bed is a big NO-NO! Your digestive system needs some kind of a break at night. It needs the rest to process everything you ingested throughout the day. Even though the body is quite fast at digesting most of the food you eat, it still needs time to detoxify and get rid of some of the chemicals and reset cortisol levels to get ready for the next day. Spending the night digesting will just slow it down and impair its ability to regenerate and produce natural growth hormones to speed up the fat loss process.

To support the fact that the meat and nuts breakfast helps support your blood sugar positively throughout the day, look at what most people call the "afternoon crash." If the first thing you put in your mouth in the morning is sugary foods or higher glycemic index foods such as refined sugar cereals, breads and/or bagels, which triggers more insulin than your body can handle, you engage your body in a freaky energy roller-coaster ride.

The ability to control your blood sugar lies in your hands. There is a growing belief that the less insulin you produce in your lifetime, the longer you'll live. Don't get me wrong, you will always produce some insulin whether you like it or not. Without going into details, here's a great way to understand insulin resistance and blood sugar.

Let's say you want to fill up a small glass of water. If you open a fire hydrant to fill up a small glass of water, it could get messy. So for those having a shitload of simple carbohydrates in a day, the sugar is the water of the fire hydrant, and the glass is what you can actually tolerate as sugar or carbohydrates. So what is left outside the glass is excess sugar floating around in your blood, some of which is eventually transformed to stored fat.

This is exactly what needs to be mastered: the ability to control your insulin. The only way to do it is to eat a good balance of simple and complex carbohydrates at every meal. In other words, seasonal fruits and all sorts of vegetables will have a better impact on your body than a candy bar.

The meat and nuts breakfast does just that, creating a minimal insulin response, since the meal consists only of protein and fats. However, if you can eat a portion of veggies in the morning, it is a plus. For those who can't have nuts due to allergies, I would suggest eating some other type of fat such as avocado, just plain veggies or a small portion of fruits like berries. Don't forget to rotate your meat, veggies and nuts at every meal. Never eat the same thing over and over again. This can lead to some food intolerance.

Habit #2: Moving often and getting stronger

One of the main focuses of the elite samurai and modern-day soldiers is to move often and stay strong. They practice their arts every single day and also take their health seriously, so any habits you will read about here, they have followed.

Hence, it goes without saying that one of the best habits to have is to be active. I get often asked if just playing a sport is good enough. My answer will be yes but only for a short while. The body is a very good, well-oiled machine. Once the body gets used to a stress, it will adapt to it. Whether this is psychological or physical, it will adapt. Being physically fit has many advantages and reflects on every aspect of our lives. However, being physically fit needs a new definition, as everyone has their own. I am not against any type of physical activity, as you must love what you are doing. Unfortunately, some habits have to match the rest of the lifestyle.

I will not ask you to go to the gym four times a week. If you have a hard time fitting in two sessions. I will not ask you to run 30 minutes day when your body is telling you to slow down and rest your adrenals. I believe we all have a life, and the constant search for balance will always be a quest. With thousands of people who have come in my office, one of the most beneficial ways to get them in shape was with weightlifting or strength training. Why?

- It's not stressful.
- We were designed to be strong.

- You can benefit from sessions of only 30 minutes.
- It improves your posture.
- It is a stress reliever.
- It helps lower cortisol levels.
- It increases metabolism.
- Lean muscle mass makes you burn fat more efficiently.

Let's keep it simple. How do you know how much is good for you and whether you should do less or do more? Here is my take on it. If you are stressed and wired or tired out and can't (or won't) do something about it, I wouldn't suggest that you train more. If stress is an issue, stay at two to three days a week, until you manage, or want to do something about it. I hope this book will help you out and give you the necessary tools. Lifestyle changes and supplements are a must if you want to do more. Keep reading, help is on the way.

Now for those of you who can tolerate or manage stress and your lifestyle efficiently, I strongly suggest that you bump up your workouts from three to four or five days a week. There are so many ways you can change your workouts and add some great things to them to make them more interesting. Look at what your goals are and change them accordingly. For example, you can add an energy system work to your routine without necessarily adding more exercises in your workout protocol. Keep your weightlifting program a three-day split, including but not limited to torso, legs, and arms, and in the remaining two days, you can add some tabata/energy system workouts and some strongman-style workouts.

The point is to train with weights and not to be afraid of building strength and lean muscle mass. This suggestion is as good for females as it is for males. No one ever became a bodybuilder from one week to the next. Train for the time you have. If you have 30 minutes a day and three days a week to devote to your workout, so be it. It's better that than nothing at all.

Cause and effect: LAZINESS, plain and simple. Most people don't want to get out of their comfortable zone. They have more excuses than a pregnant nun. However, the most common excuse is lack of energy. To a certain point, we can blame it on the current diet, so in all fairness, give yourself a week or two with habit number one, which is the meat and nuts breakfast, and you should start seeing a difference in your energy level. The problem is that, afterwards, you may have no excuse for not working out!

Lack of time? Worst excuse ever. Even a little bout of exercise daily has many benefits. Some people may not have time to get to the gym, or they are just busy at home taking care of the kids. A small investment can go a long way. For about the same price as a gym membership, you can get yourself a great home gym, with many toys you can play around with. For example, many of my beginners who don't have time to get to the gym invested in a Swiss ball, free weights and a special attachment like the Tower 200, which requires only a doorframe. These are equipped for a full year of training. The Tower 200 works like a pulley system, but with elastics. A good trainer can get the most out of this type of equipment and can at least get you started, with a good little workout that fills up a small part of your busy schedule.

The bottom line is to stay active. As soon as you stop moving, the body deteriorates and eats itself up. It's as simple as that.

Habit #3: Getting your sleep right

It's all a matter of quality. If you can't sleep a full night without waking up, then you may want to look into it. However, sleeping for more than nine hours a night may also be a problem. Sometimes more is not better. Every time I ask the question, "Are you sleeping well?" most people say they are. Beauty is in the eye of the beholder. Great sleep means different things to different people. In my practice, I would estimate that one out of three clients has had or is having some kind of sleep disturbance. As a matter of fact, hours slept per night on average have greatly decreased in the past 50 years. A 1960s survey of one million people found that the average number of hours slept per night was eight to nine hours. In 2000, the average decreased to about seven hours. Currently, the average has further declined to about five or six hours of sleep.

The major player in disturbed sleep patterns is the hormone cortisol. Cortisol, which is secreted by the adrenal glands, is involved in several important functions including, glucose metabolism, regulation of blood pressure, insulin release for blood sugar maintenance, immune function and inflammatory response. Although performing some significant functions, we must remember that our bodies are not designed to endure long periods of stress, which, needless to say, is a symptom of our society.

When levels of cortisol are elevated for an extended period of time, the following symptoms become prevalent:

- Impaired cognitive performance;
- Suppressed thyroid function;
- Blood sugar imbalances such as hyperglycemia;
- Decreased bone density;
- Decrease in muscle tissue;
- Higher blood pressure;
- Lowered immunity and inflammatory responses in the body, slowed wound healing and
- other health consequences;
- Increased abdominal fat, which is associated with a greater number of health problems such as heart attacks, strokes or the development of metabolic syndrome.

Another major worry that I often encounter in my practice is overtraining, which puts a stress on the adrenal glands that are responsible for the release and elevated levels of cortisol in the body. When training for prolonged periods of time, our body is in a constant state of stimulus, which it portrays as stress. We become chronically stimulated, or hyper-stimulated. When we are constantly hyper-stimulated, we can't sleep, and the sleep we are getting is not as restful.

If an external stress prevents you from sleeping, than treat it accordingly. In addition, you must examine your lifestyle and/or stress levels. Sleep disturbance is induced. It does not occur without cause. Although it may start slowly it can easily get worse, affecting simple things like **weight management.** The release of hormones by the pituitary – the "master" endocrine organ that controls the secretion of other hormones from the peripheral endocrine glands – is markedly influenced by sleep. Modulation of pituitary-dependent hormonal release is partly mediated by the modulation of the activity of hypothalamic-releasing and/or hypothalamic-inhibiting factors controlling pituitary function. During sleep, these hypothalamic factors may be activated, as in the case of growth hormone (GH)-releasing hormone. When sleep deprivation is prevalent, it promotes the development of insulin resistance, which is closely related to obesity and diabetes.

Research has shown that animals subjected to sleep loss for prolonged periods of time were more likely to have an increase in appetite. Studies in humans have shown that the levels of hormones that regulate appetite are greatly influenced by sleep disturbance. Sleep loss is linked with an increase in appetite that is disproportionate in relation to the caloric load of extensive wakefulness. In other words, you are up and awake longer, so you obviously eat more while awake. Recent work also indicates that sleep loss may harmfully affect glucose tolerance and may be involved in an increased risk of Type 2 diabetes. In young, healthy subjects who were studied after six days of sleep restriction (four hours in bed) and after full sleep recovery, the levels of blood glucose after breakfast were higher in the state of sleep debt despite normal or even slightly elevated insulin responses. The difference in peak glucose levels in response to breakfast averaged ±15 mg/dL, a difference large enough for a significant impairment of glucose tolerance. These results were established by the results of intravenous glucose tolerance testing. Indeed, the rate of disappearance of glucose post injection, a quantitative measure of glucose tolerance, was nearly 40% slower in the sleep-debt condition than after recovery, and the acute insulin response to glucose was reduced by 30%.

Let's quit the technical mumbo-jumbo and skip to what everyone wants to know: how do I deal with all this? My answer would be to define your greatest concern and deal with it. The following are some ways to maybe discover some possible concerns, but are not methods for diagnosis. If any health concerns are looming, please, do not hesitate to consult with your general practitioner. See the following as some tools to maybe help you identify some greater problems coming your way if you don't look into it. Let's look at some of the **misfires** some of you may have.

1.Difficulty falling asleep

Mostly the result of elevated cortisol at night: If you have a hard time falling asleep, or just can't get to relax at night, high night-time cortisol is usually a problem. If you took care of all the bad late-night habits mentioned previously, than you should look at other types of solutions such as magnesium. Magnesium deficiency affects as much as 70% of the population, and I've never seen someone with optimal levels, all the more so if you are a training advocate, since exercise depletes magnesium levels. Besides the fact that it is involved in over 300 enzymatic reactions in our bodies, it also helps your muscles relax and is great at inducing sleep at night.. I usually use ubermag or ubermag plus from the Poliquin brand. Both are the same except that the ubermag plus has L-Tryptophan in it, which is a greater sleep inducer. Ubermag is made from a mixture of magnesium chelates, which are better absorbed by the body.

- Magnesium Fumerate is an intermediate of the Krebs cycle, which plays a part in energy production in human physiological systems.
- Magnesium orotate helps cardiovascular health.
- Magnesium glycinate helps the liver detoxify.
- Magnesium taurate is calming and increases the happy neurotransmitter, GABA.

2. Difficulty staying asleep

Your liver might be the one who is waking you up. It is saying that something is not right, some food intolerance or some sub-optimal kind of detoxification is going on when it tries to wake you up in the middle of the night. Liver detox protocol and some anti-oxidants are in order. I would suggest that you consult your nearest bio-signature practitioners for a good and thorough consultation and evaluation. Please do not use over-the-counter detox products as they most often contain some kind of preservatives such as parabens, which defeats the whole purpose of the detox.

3. Difficulty waking up.

Low morning cortisol: Usual symptoms are difficulty getting up, morning brain fog, irritability and low overall energy throughout the day, with the usual crash around 3 p.m. I found that eating late is one of the main reasons why someone could have a hard time waking up in the morning, but if late-night snacks are not in the equation, low morning cortisol is usually a bigger problem. A natural way to bring up low morning cortisol is to drink a full glass of water with a pinch of sea salt. After a couple of days, morning cortisol levels should be back up to normal. If you want to use supplements, which are probably a better solution, I use licorice in the morning. It extends the half-life of cortisol, and at the same time it brings back normal cortisol levels throughout the day as well.

4. All of the above

Cortisol flat liners: Those are the ones that, no matter what they do, can't get results. No matter how hard they push or how well they eat, they will always be stuck at the same weight, with some very small highs and lows. This is not something to be taken lightly, because the cause is adrenal exhaustion, or what is commonly known as adrenal fatigue syndrome. Here are the usual symptoms: fatigue, lethargy, lack of energy in the morning and also in the afternoon between 3 p.m. and 5 p.m., fatigue between

9 p.m. and 10 p.m. but resistance to going to bed, light-headed-ness (including dizziness and fainting) when rising from a sitting or prone position, lowered blood pressure and blood sugar, diffi-culty concentrating or remembering (brain fog), consistently feel-ing unwell or difficulty recovering from infections, craving either salty or sugary foods to keep going, unexplained hair loss, nausea, alternating constipation and diarrhea, mild depression, decreased sex drive, sleep difficulties, unexplained pain in the upper back or neck, increased PMS symptoms among women (periods are heavy and then stop or almost stop on the fourth day only to start again on the fifth or sixth day), tendency to gain weight and inability to lose it (especially around the waist), and high frequency of getting the flu and other respiratory diseases, plus a tendency for them to last longer than usual.

As you may have seen, symptoms do not vary greatly from one condition to another, but flat liners are the ones that will always keep on until they crash, and when they crash, it's for a very long time, followed by a major illness or disease. The main cause of adrenal fatigue is the inability to see previous signs of fatigue or disturbed cortisol signals. In my world, it is also called overtraining. I have a very simple test I use to determine if one of my athletes is in overtraining; it's called the grip test. I mea-sure their grip with a dynamometer first thing in the morning. When the values go down, it means that overtraining is starting to settle in. It does not mean that I send them home, but I can at least adjust their training accordingly and give them the rest they need. When adrenal fatigue is inevitable, I use Cordicep

Mycellum and Rhodiola Rosea. It is a specially formulated herbal combination that gives a boost to the adrenals when they are down and out, and calms them when they are stressed out of their minds.

Late night habit #1: Working late

This is not for those of you who are working on shifts or the night shifts: that's a whole different matter. I'm talking about those of you who come home as usual between 5 p.m. and 7 p.m., have dinner, go out a bit or take care of the spouse and kids, and when everybody is asleep, go back on the laptop, and finish the day's work, answer some emails, or whatever work needs to be done for the following day. The problem is that, as soon as you open the screen, your eyes can perceive the light of the screen as it would with daylight. Before going to bed, you should dim the lights, relax, and not think about anything except maybe what went well today, and think of how you should improve tomorrow. Working prior to bed keeps your cortisol level up when it should be going down. I already hear you say that work needs to be done, but look into your personal time management schedule. You have one, don't you? If not, divide your day in advance, knowing what's going to happen (approximately), and I'm sure you'll find some time you could be doing work instead of looking at Facebook or answering emails that can wait. Planning your day in advance is the key. My first advice to you is to go to bed earlier, but wake up early. Working, studying or training when you are fresh and rested will bring better results.

Late night habit #2: Eating late

Another bad habit that I see too often is eating late or too close to bedtime. Our body is made for regeneration at night, so eating prior to your Z's delays this process to a certain extent. If you sleep properly, every hormone is set into place to help your body regenerate properly and be ready for the next day or for challenges. But if you eat something that puts your digestive system to the test, your liver and enzymes will only focus on trying to process your late meal instead of resting and preparing for the next day to come.

Late night habit #3: TV, news or arguments before bed

Although it could be categorized together with habit #1, this is different for one simple reason: it's more likely a personal choice, not driven by work or unfinished business. People often think they can fall asleep in front of the television or that watching a movie will help them relax. More often than not, TV will help you stay awake the same way your laptop or computer will. First things first, TVs are getting bigger and bigger, not to mention surround-sound systems. Movies are not a bad idea, but looking at Jason Statham kick some ass at lightning speed can't possibly help bring your cortisol down and may well bring it up. Maybe some boring old documentary could do the trick, but to be proactive, why not learn something at the same time and read a good book under dimmed light to help induce your sleep?

One of the best ways that I often practice myself and strongly suggest to clients and friends is to do a grateful log, which I learned from my mentors. I do a quick run-up of what went **well** in the day, no matter how bad the day was. This helps me to put my mind in a positive state prior to bed. You don't want to start thinking about all negative stuff to get your mind racing.

Here is an example of one of my good friend and fellow strength coach Ryan from <u>Enfuse Fitness</u>.

1. *Very productive day. I am grateful I was able to get a lot done, enabling us to move forward.*
2. *My buddy Joey caught me off guard. He knows I've had a bit going on and just reached out to see how I was doing and to let me know he was thinking of me. That meant a lot! Thanks brother!*
3. *I baby-sat Ty and Lili's pups so they could have a date night! ENJOY, GUYS!*
4. *I had to reschedule the nature walk because people are worried about the weather (understandably so with a potential hurricane). So I am excited about doing it one day next week when the weather will be beautiful!*

Even when things are going sucky, you can easily turn that thought around and put it into your grateful log. The idea is to put your mind into a positive state and bring all your thoughts on paper. Setting all your possible problems aside will eliminate night-time mind racing and will help you wake up with a good fresh mental state, ready to tackle the next day.

Cortisol is something we need, but like everything in life, when in excess, it can do more harm than good. With today's stress levels and longer work hours, we need to take care of our health, more than ever before. If you think you are superman and want to do a thousand things at the same time, without proper rest, it will catch up to you, one day or another. Being able to recognize the early sign of sleep disturbance is the key. Don't wait until it gets worse and focus on recharging your batteries before more problems occur.

Habit #4: Staying away from man-made food

This must be one of your absolute priorities. If you have followed the meat and nuts breakfast and followed through with nutrition plans such as the Paleolithic or Mediterranean diets, you must have felt it by now, that eating as closely as possible to our ancestors will help us lead a healthy life. Jack Lalanne said it best: if man made it, don't eat it.

The reasons for eliminating these food choices are pretty obvious. There will always be those diehard dairy cheese and yogurt fans, who in reality are more afraid of letting go of their little comfort food rather than of changing their nutrition habits. Those who don't have time for breakfast or can't be talked out of their peanut butter and toast in the morning are probably those who would pull a fit if you tried to change their morning ritual. They will fight to the death before they even start considering changing these food choices. However, EVERYONE who did make the switch had great results. Better digestion, lost inches on their stomachs, lost body fat, better skin, concentration, etc. I dare you to try.

Even our veggies are labeled man-made. Man intoxicates them, to produce more and do it faster. To make sure they don't lose money with wasted crops, they will go the extra mile, even if they are not sure whether certain chemicals could be potentially hazardous to consumers' health. If there is no potential danger to our health, why do they spray with full chemical suits on? The use of pesticides is destroying all the nutrients and wreaks havoc on our ecosystem. Even though the U.S. Department of Agriculture constantly tries to make us believe that pesticides are safe and there is no proof of toxicity, I call this (and we should all) bullshit for money.

"A group of three long-term studies found that a woman's exposure to organophosphate pesticides during pregnancy could affect IQ and memory in her child six to nine years later. Researchers at Mount Sinai School of Medicine, University of California Berkeley's School of Public Health and Columbia University's Mailman School of Public Health separately recruited pregnant women and tested either their mother's urine during pregnancy or umbilical blood at birth. All three studies are available free and online at the Environmental Health Perspectives website. And you can hear it for yourself on ABC's World News Tonight." — Taken from the Environmental Working Group blog.

Even canned food, regarded as a better alternative, is a big problem. The insides are coated with a plastic shield, protecting us from some residues of the can, but this plastic contains BPA (Bisphenol A), which is highly toxic.

- A study showed that BPA exposure leads to a cell division error called aneuploidy that causes spontaneous miscarriages, cancer and birth defects in people, including Downs Syndrome (Hunt et al. 2003).
- An investigation demonstrating that low doses of BPA spur both the formation and growth of fat cells, the two factors that drive obesity in humans (Masumo et al. 2002).
- A study linking low doses of BPA to insulin resistance, a risk factor for Type 2 diabetes (Alonso-Magdalena et al. 2006).
- A preliminary investigation linking BPA exposures to recurrent miscarriage in a small group of Japanese women, made potentially pivotal by its concordance with lab studies of BPA-induced chromosome damage that could well cause miscarriage (Sugiura-Ogasawara 2005).

The goal is to shop clean and avoid these chemicals as much as we can. If you can't, just do your best: it's better than nothing. Buy lean meats from a butcher you know and who, if possible, buys and sells free-range and can have access to some tall-grass-fed beef or wild game. Clean your veggies before eating them and buy them organic as much as possible. The return on your investment won't be visible, but you'll see it in the long run with fewer health problems for you and your family. Pay organic farmers now or pay for meds later in life.

Have you ever stepped back and look at what is sold at the supermarket? Look at the majority of the food they sell. More than 80% of store food is man-made. There are whole aisles reserved for breads, cereals, cookies, snacks, soft drinks and other beverages and TV dinners. That is man-made food at its most obvious, anything to do with wheat and sugar and anything that has to be mixed and baked in order to be eaten.

The number one rule when someone steps in my office is to cut out all kinds of man-made food, such as those mentioned above. Why? They contain all kinds of sugar, preservatives and gluten. For example, artificial sweeteners are in almost every beverage, except, you guessed it, pure water. It's no secret that soft drinks and sugar are the major culprit of today's obesity pandemic. They are the main reason for the rise in cases of Type 2 diabetes, high blood pressure and heart disease. Then there are those who will go for the sugar-free and fat-free options. How can something be sugar-free and still taste sweet? If it looks like shit and tastes like shit, it must be shit, right? Although some research tries to prove that this may be a solution to the obesity pandemic, more and more research proves this theory wrong, showing that it may be part of the problem. National health and nutritional surveys have clearly noted the association between increased intake of these so-called natural sweeteners and obesity, high cholesterol, elevated blood pressure and glucose. Another study done on rats proved that, when artificial sweeteners were added to their normal chow, they consumed more food and gained more weight.

Nothing is really clear why this can occur, but it may have to do with the fact that it disrupts our normal appetite patterns and blunts how our bodies can manage glucose and insulin. In 1958, two sweeteners by the name of saccharin and cyclamate were labeled as safe by governments, which went back on their word 20 years later because of worries over cancer risks linked to these two chemicals. Another sweetener to look out for is aspartame. Experiments have proved that it may induce cancer, damage DNA and trigger major migraines. It has been shown that aspartame triggers migraine in some cases because it gets broken down into methanol and AKA wood alcohol, in our bodies. Although I did not find any conclusive research on the damage leading to elevated levels of methanol but who cares, it's still methanol and it's still toxic.

Another problem is gluten, which is used more than you think and even hidden. Linked to celiac disease and all kinds of degenerative health issues, it is in my opinion the silent killer of the 21st century. Some symptoms are very mild but, in the long run, it can damage your digestive system in many ways. Nothing explains better the impact that man has had on how we change the genetic makeup of our food than this excerpt from an interview with Dr. William Davis on the evils of wheat.

"Comparing a conventional wheat plant from 50 years ago against a modern high-yield dwarf wheat plant, you would see that today's plant is about 2½ feet shorter. It's stockier, so it can support a much heavier seedbed, and it grows much faster. The great irony here is that the term 'genetic modification' refers to the actual insertion or deletion of a gene, and that's not what's happened with wheat. Instead, the plant has been hybridized and crossbred to make it resistant to drought and fungi, and to vastly increase yield per acre. Agricultural geneticists have shown that wheat proteins undergo structural change with hybridization and that the hybrid contains proteins that are found in neither parent plant. Now, it shouldn't be the case that every single new agricultural hybrid has to be checked and tested, that would be absurd. But we've created thousands of what I call Frankengrains over the past 50 years, using pretty extreme techniques, and their safety for human consumption has never been tested or even questioned."

Need I say more?

Got Milk?

I find it pretty amusing when I see celebrities sell their name and attach it to the "Got Milk?" campaign, when it is pretty obvious that the last thing in their mind is drinking milk. What does this have to do with man-made food? Doesn't milk come from a cow? No shit, Sherlock! But what I would like to know is who got the idea, or when did someone think, that we could drink the white liquid that comes out of a cow's dangling part? More and more, we see people with some kind of lactose intolerance and allergies that come out of nowhere. There are problems with the milk we drink. It's a fact that American milk is banned in Europe because it is genetically modified. They inject rBGH in cows to make them produce more and faster. However, rBGH increases cancer risks. There is also the undeniable fact that 65% of all milk drinkers experiences gas, bloating and digestive distress. The rest can probably tolerate dairy products better because they maintain a higher level of the enzyme lactase in their gut, so they can metabolize lactose without experiencing bouts of gas and stomach discomfort. The impact it has on insulin is also a concern. Despite the fact that most dairy products have a low glycemic index, they have a high insulin response similar to white bread. So it is a big no-no for those with insulin resistance, contrary to popular belief.

Take a look or Google some of these research and papers on why milk is not the best option.
Dangers of IGF-1 in Milk include Breast, Colon and Prostate Cancers
Cancer Risks from IGF-1. Monsanto's Hormonal Milk
Breast Cancer Risks from rBGH (Press Conference)
Colon and Breast Cancer Risks from rBGH (Press Conference)
Prostate Cancer Risks from IGF-1 press release
FDA allows rBGH to endanger Milk
United Nations ban on rBGH, Monsanto's Genetically Modified Milk
Scientific Article on rBGH (1990) "Potential Public Health Hazards of Biosynthetic Milk Hormones"

Scientific Article on IGF-1 (1996) "Unlabeled Milk from Cows Treated with Biosynthetic Growth Hormones"

Why would you take a chance and eat something that can damage your quest to leanness and maybe even your health? Yes, you can indulge once in a while, but there are always better alternatives. Stay with the organic and natural stuff.

> *"The body is like a revolver, and the toxins/chemicals we put in it are the bullets.*
> *Every time you expose your body to those toxins and chemicals, you load up a bullet. One day you wake up and life pulls the trigger."*
> — *Mark Schauss*

Habit #5: Using your head

Take 30 minutes a day to do something new, or work on a new project that has been put on hold, whether work-related or not.

This one does not look very productive, and one would think that it could set you back in your current occupations. This could not be further from the truth. All you may need is to take your mind out of what you're doing five days a week (more like seven days a week) and try something new. We all have those crazy ideas of inventing or creating something that can make our lives easier. Did you ever think about doing something that sounded too crazy to do, and that made people think you were nuts?

Tell that to the freak who invented "Snuggies." They look like KKK robes minus the hat, but you know what, that guy sold 25 million of them. HE ONLY PUT SLEEVES ON A FREAKIN' BLANKET!!!. **The Clapper.** Clap your hands and a light goes on and off? Yes, it seems nuts to me too, but millions of people have purchased them. The person who cashes in on this idea is chanting "clap on" every time he goes to the bank!

Doing something new wakes up the creative part of the brain. Every single day we do what we know best, without challenging our grey matter. We stay in our comfortable zone and as soon as we get out of it, we look for the nearest exit to bring us back to our routine. Routine is a good thing: it keeps us from doing stupid things, but maybe this is what we need to do to learn and to challenge our minds. Getting out of our nine-to-five routine by creating a new hobby or a new passion can give us enough of a break to relax our minds and perform better in any given task when the time comes. One of the best examples I can give you is Richard Branson. If you don't know who he is, you just found something new to do. Read his book, Losing My Virginity.

"My interest in life comes from setting myself huge, apparently unachievable challenges and trying to rise above them ... from the perspective of wanting to live life to the full, I felt that I had to attempt it."

Habit #6: Being grateful

Be grateful. Gratitude precludes envy and greed, cures anger, heals resentment, encourages a sense of contentment and promotes moderation, restraint and balance. Good health is what you owe to yourself but also for the world around you. Be grateful for your parents and nature itself that gives you all you need to sustain life. The highest ingratitude of all towards your parents and towards the society that educated and provided for you is to neglect your health.

Habit #7: Healing the not yet ill

Like in the 5 warrior habits seen at the beginning, winning the battle before it even begins is best. Using your resources skillfully will avoid great and dangerous battles. Most people don't think or are not in touch enough with their body, which gives them signals of possible problems coming their way like a cold or insomnia like seen in habit number three. This is the way you should use Yojokun, committing yourself to being victorious (healthy) before the battle even begins (illness). Prevention is the key.

Habit #8: Using your time wisely

Although I've read all kinds of ways to improve time management, there is no better way to deal with a lack of time than to take out time and energy wasters. There is always the positive list where what you think will become useful but sometimes reminding us that what slows us down is a need to get back on track. We all know our weaknesses, but ignoring them just makes them more powerful since it is easy to succumb to temptation. This goes against most lifestyle management or positive thinking programs, but these programs do not work for everybody.

Make a "not to do" list, as a reminder of what not to do in your day. Don't go on Facebook or Twitter while working, don't miss a meal, don't work late, don't forget to drink plenty of water, etc. Every single thing that you spend time doing while you know you shouldn't are things that can easily be stopped, but procrastination holds you back. Do you want that promotion more than you want to keep on chatting on Facebook? You decide.

Another big problem is that we must learn to say no. We have to prioritize and take chances, follow our gut instinct and choose tasks that we know we can do effectively. Saying no to deals we know will set us back or just put us down is, in my opinion, a no-brainer.

Once you get rid of the so-called time wasters, attack your top priorities first. Here's a little story to illustrate my point. A teacher puts a small fish tank on the desk and starts by putting big rocks in them. "Is the tank full?" he asks. Most of the students reply no. Obviously, it wasn't, so he starts to put pebbles in the tank, filling the space between the big rocks. Then he asks again if the tank was full. A majority of the students reply yes. He starts pouring some sand to fill the space between the big rocks and the pebbles. Then he asks again if the tank was full. Everybody says yes, but at the same time he starts to pour water in the tank. Then he says, "Now the tank is full!" Following that, he empties everything and repeats the same exercise by putting the water first, followed by the sand and pebbles. When it was time to put the rocks in the tank, there was no more space left.

What's the lesson of the story? Start with your top priorities and everything will fall into place. If you sweat the small stuff, your important priorities will always be set aside. Plan your week ahead of time; place your big rocks first. On Sunday night, decide what would have to be done in the following week. This would work not only with your business: be sure to include tasks that could help you achieve personal goals or lifelong dreams. For example, if you want to improve your body composition, one goal would be to eat at least one source of protein five to six times a day. Preparing all your food in advance would help you achieve this goal. Start with "five big rocks" per week, about one a day. Judging by how you deal with these commitments, you'll improve your ability to put in more big rocks as you go along. If you're on a schedule, make sure your "big rocks" are included as part of it. Try and schedule them with associated tasks so that you know you'll be able to achieve them. Give yourself enough time to do it, not between busy times or meetings. Remember, big rocks are best done first thing in the morning. Tasks can easily get pushed aside, so doing them early will leave space for less important work. When the week is done, look back at it and acknowledge your success at getting them done.

Habit #9: Early to bed, early to rise

It really does make you healthy and wise, for many reasons. Some people need six hours of sleep and others won't start to be functional unless they get at least nine hours, and so it all depends on individual needs. My advice would be to go to bed before 11 p.m. and to get up at around 6 a.m. or 7 a.m.

The problem with sleeping in is that it screws up your schedule. For example, if I were to suggest that to lose fat, you needed to get at least four meals a day, doing so would be almost impossible since you just skipped breakfast. A regular feeding schedule would have you eat your first meal of the day at around 6 or 7 o'clock in the morning, with regular meals every three or four hours, finishing with your last meal at 7 p.m. Skipping breakfast will leave you with only three meals. Yes, this is not the end of the world, but it has been proven that those who tend to forego the first meal of the day have higher levels of Leptin, a hormone that plays a key role in regulating energy intake and expenditure, including hunger and metabolism. Before you think that this is to compensate for the amount of calories lost in the first meal, it has a much more damaging impact than eating five equally balanced meals at regular intervals.

First, the higher calorie count will leave you full and maybe create a negative impact on your insulin and fat-burning abilities. Next will be the cravings at night. They will often be uncontrollable. Last but not least, if you succumbed to your cravings, instead of resting and regenerating while sleeping as intended, your body will spend he night digesting and impairing your ability to rest and to detoxify, produce growth hormones and regenerate, thus impairing again your ability to burn fat.

Most businessmen I work with will bring work home with them at night to be done once the kids are asleep or just to do when they have time, usually before bed. One of the worst things they can do is to bring their computers to work on in bed. First, the light of the laptop will have the same effect as daylight, which will mix up the signal and tell your body to wake up. Next is the fact that the heat from the laptop will cook your eggs, a.k.a. testies, a.k.a. your balls, which lowers sperm count, among other problems.

Cause and effect: Never work before bedtime. It only wakes you up more and will make your sleep quality miserable. My advice would be to go to bed early and mentally rested and then to wake up earlier to do your work, while having a wholesome breakfast. Your rested mind and energy will make you more productive, and your morning coffee will always be of great help. You'll also be sure to have your early breakfast full of protein to boost your dopamine levels and to increase your neurotransmitters to take on the day's work.

Habit #10: Emptying your glass

We all like to watch movies or read a good book. Go out for lunch with friends or just spend time with your loved ones. We mostly do this because we enjoy it, but for some it is a good way to forget things, ease our minds, forget our problems and just let go. When was the last time you sit or lay down and just thought about nothing, nada, niet, nothing at all? While awake? This is called meditation. Before you jump straight to the next habit, just take a few moments to finish reading this. When people think or hear about meditation, they suddenly think about Gandhi, in his MC hammer white pants sitting on a carpet with a smell of wooden incense. He suddenly starts flying around on the incense's clouds and start talking about life and our purpose on earth. Let me snap you back into reality for a moment. Meditation is a way to empty your mind and make peace with yourself. Meditation is mostly a self-centered moment, happening quietly in your own head. Some people may do it lying down or sitting on a bench alone in a park. You can even do it in your bath. You don't have to achieve monk level 10 in order to meditate. Just do some soul searching.

Here is what can happen in your mind while meditating. Look for emptiness. How can you do that? Let go of any thoughts you have in your mind by visualizing yourself emptying a big wooden crate. As you empty the crate, thought by thought, it seems that the crate is becoming bigger and bigger, and you will suddenly find yourself in an empty state of mind, visualizing yourself floating around as if in space, in that giant wooden crate that you call your head. I know some who visualize a big desk with endless drawers, which they open up and clean up until they have put everything, all their thoughts, in the last drawer, the garbage.

This is only one example of how to visualize your trip north. Find your peace within. However, you must empty your thinking box, from this moment on, to make way for positive thoughts.

Misfires: You can't think straight? You get frustrated over nothing? Stress levels keep going higher and higher? There is a close link between magnesium deficiency and anxiety. Since magnesium is involved in over 300 chemical processes in the body, being deficient is really not a good thing. One of the advantages of having proper magnesium levels is improved memory.

Magnesium increases brain function by improving electrical activity, thus increasing learning abilities and memory functions. It also has an impact on depression-like symptoms. In addition, it helps release serotonin, one of the feel-good hormones.

Habit #11 Choosing your surroundings wisely

You are the mirror of whom you most hang around with. They will affect your attitude, energy, thoughts and emotional state, whether you like it or not. Let's say you decide to take your health in charge, except that your friends are the complete opposite. Look at Mary the lawyer, my good friend in the examples earlier in this book. A major challenge for her was some of her friends. Don't get me wrong: changing friends is not the easiest thing to do, and it sounds really conceited, but the reality is that some of them may be, and let's be realistic here, amazing losers. If you are familiar with the Saturday Night Live sketch "Debbie Downer," it is a very good look at some friends who literally drain your energy because of their unbelievably negative babbling.

One of my worst enemies is, more often than not, people's surroundings and immediate family. Believe it or not, there are some people who don't want others to succeed. Today's society wants the best with the least effort. When they see someone succeed through hard work and dedication, they find ways to criticize or degrade that person's results and efforts. Their primary goal is to bring people down to their level.

What to do: It is your life and goals. You will never see successful people hang around losers, so do the same. You can always talk to some of your less than positive friends and let them know that you have a goal and that you need all the help you can get. If you see that with their attitude that they seem receptive and are genuine about their intent of helping you, that is a true friend. If not, you know what is left to do. Just to reassure you, every person that I know who made a little "cleanup" in his or her surroundings saw only improvement afterwards. Reaching their goals was a lot easier too.

Habit #12: Chewing your food wisely

This one seems so obvious you would think that everybody does it. If only it were that simple. For example, most people have a hard time eating breakfast because they are in such a hurry. Imagine taking the time to sit down and eat in a relaxed state. Those who eat properly in the morning while reading the paper and sipping on their coffee have a much better chance of fat loss and having a great day than those who eat on the edge of the table while multitasking the whole family in the morning.

There are also business lunches where you eat slowly, too slowly, because of the never-ending conversations and poor service at the restaurant. However, even though the goal is to eat slowly and chew properly, you always seem to feel bloated after those business lunches. The problem is that eating while doing business is not suggested. Even though it is some kind of way to bring clients out and thank them for their business, it is also a way to overeat and ignore your diet. Some executives I train are shy about just eating a little salad and some meat to follow their plans because they think clients will see this as a weakness. I tell them to screw what other people think: they are not the ones getting their asses kicked at my training sessions. I also never understood the requirement to eat a large unhealthy portion of fried calamari in order to get a deal. If the client wants to eat what he wants, so be it. Stop imagining that he will think less of you because you eat properly. Then again, it all depends where you eat. Even when stuck eating junk, there is one trick that will help you digest and won't set you back on your goals: **you need to CHEW your food!**

Eating in a fast and stressed manner is the best way to have digestive problems. The more stress you have, the less digestive enzymes you secrete. It's as simple as that. Sub-optimal digestion is the best way to invite problems such as stomach ulcers, constipation, leaky gut, irritable bowel syndrome, sleep apnea, etc. So recall those big business lunches and the bloating sensation after the meal, the arguing at the supper table, eating your lunch at the edge of the corner because you are pressed for time – all these situations that we often repeat are causing setbacks in our diets as well as digestive discomfort.

Eating while sitting down and taking your time to appreciate your meal is the best way to secrete enzymes and to also maximize digestion. Your mama always told you that you need to chew at least seven times before swallowing, and she was absolutely right. You have to realize that digestion starts in the mouth as well. Saliva helps by secreting salivary lipase to start breaking down fat and amylase to break down starch into sugar. It also contains antimicrobial enzymes that kill bacteria such as lysozyme, salivary lactoperoxidase, lactoferrin and immunoglobulin A. Take your time and enjoy your time when you eat, and chew until the food is almost liquid. It takes a little time for your stomach to feel that it is satisfied, so take your time. That way, overeating won't be a concern. Just by taking the habit of chewing and eating slowly, you will feel your digestion improving tremendously, and you may find that you won't need to take the HCI and/or enzymes after your meal.

If you think you don't have time in the morning, or if business lunches are inevitable, use this simple habit at every meal. You won't mess up your goals, and you'll see a huge difference. It is a small sacrifice for better gut health.

Honorable mention
Planning your perfect day

How you start and finish your day has everything to do with your quality of life. Have you ever got up in the morning and bumped your little toe against the corner of the table? How was the rest of your day? According to what people say, it's the mirror of what happened in the morning, disastrous, blaming everything on the fact that you got up on the wrong foot. Then if the day was a disaster, if you lost some important papers or messed up everything in a very important presentation, you got home, almost depressed and all you wanted was to crawl under the covers without ever waking up. The problem is that you aren't able to stop your thinking box, recalling every situation that went wrong. Consequently, you lose a couple of hours of sleep because of it, and the next day is no better, leading to a snowball effect.

There will always be some of those days. A simple trick is to visualize your perfect day. What would your dream day would look like, what it would feel like to get everything going the way you would like? I am not talking about a day reminiscent of the rich and famous. I am talking about getting up in the morning and feeling like it's going to be THE day. Offers, great weather, no rush, everything going according to plan, etc. Write down what a regular day would be like in the best of worlds. Here's how I would do it in the mind of a client.

- Get up and feel refreshed, before the alarm clock.
- Can't wait to eat my bison meat with nuts and raspberries because I'm freakin' hungry
- Sit down and have spare time to eat and spend a couple of minutes with the spouse and kids before heading to work.
- Watch my kids and wife smile (priceless).
- The weather is perfect outside, with a nice fresh breeze.
- Off to the gym.
- Arm day: let's trash them like we never did before, and indeed, trashed they are.
- Some random stranger came up to me and said he noticed that my shape has improved tremendously.
- work, everyone seemed please with everything I did. I was even offered a promotion.
- Got back home, no traffic whatsoever, and a parking spot right in front of the apartment.
- Kids jumped in my arms as I walked through the door, and I got a huge hug from my spouse.

- A perfect diner was already on the table.
- Everyone pitched in to clean up after the meal so that we could have time to rest and spend the evening together.
- Kids in bed, my spouse made me a happy camper (hey, who wouldn't want to).
- Slept like a baby

Everyone is different, so go ahead and make your perfect day, and you can be as explicit as you want. You can write everything down, from feelings to smells, and use your imagination, because nothing is impossible. Keep the paper where you can see it, and look at it once in a while. You'll see that you may be closer to your perfect day than you thought you ever would be. You may be setting your perfect week and aligning everything to get what you want. Chances are that one thing will lead to another, you'll find that your life is as perfect as you desire, and you'll see yourself in total control of your day and your destiny. It's no secret that those who write down their goals are the most successful at it. Why not do the same with your perfect day

Chapter 4

Acquiring strengths

Ten years ago, my friend Stephen and I got an offer to train body-guards in South Africa. I would have taken care of the health and physical aspects of the guards, while he would take care of the com-bat and logistics. However, I was fortunate enough to be trained like them, think like them and know what they have to go through, as I was also studying to get involved and try my hand at the close protection business.

The intestinal fortitude needed to go through live scenarios is as intense as the real situation, minus the death threat. One way to acquire strength is to conquer your fears. I will walk you through some of my live training scenarios and how they helped me shape programs for future agents in training and, in the process, under-stand how we can fight our worst fears. Keep in mind that, with a stressful workload and life-threatening jobs, mental acuity is of the utmost importance, so my biggest task was to make the nutrition aspect as perfect as possible for each participant. Most of them had to be very fit prior to the actual program due to strict enrolment procedures. First and foremost, I must clarify something: this had nothing to do with the stereotype of "the bodyguard" in the movie with Kevin Costner and Whitney Houston.

The logistics behind a simple Point A to Point B VIP transport can be grueling and can be spread over several days, more so if the client is of political interest in foreign countries. For example, three assassination attempts were mounted against Eduard Shevardnadze, a former Soviet foreign minister, and later, Georgian statesman from the height to the end of the Cold War. The 1995 attack had seen his motorcade attacked with anti-tank rockets and small arms fire in Tbilisi under cover of night (Katz, Samuel M. "Relentless Pursuit: The DSS and the manhunt for the al-Qaeda terrorists," 2002). I saw footage of the attack and, let me tell you one thing, although you can never prepare for that, you must be ready at all times.

A survey of the 1998–2000 period compiled by the United Nations Office on Drugs and Crime ranked South Africa second for assault and murder (through all means) per capita and first for rapes per capita in a dataset of 60 countries. Total crime per capita was 10th out of the 60 countries in the dataset. Needless to say, this fired me up and, as one of my friends says, you need to put yourself in danger in order to move forward, so I guess I did. Besides my varied martial arts knowledge, my biggest task was the technical and tactical part of the job. I became certified with the Level 2 Monadnock PR-24 extensible baton and restraint techniques (only available for police officers) which was, by the way, very painful.

Try joint locks and restraints with a steel rod. I also got my acquisition and possession permit for firearms, target and precision shooting, which I passed with 96% alongside a guy who was in the army for many years. In that certification, I learned to use different kind of firearms, along with the tactical part such as room clearing and other situations relevant to the field. The longest but most technical part of the training was the legal part. There is a whole protocol to follow when you interrogate or when the law interrogates you if ever an incident occurs. I learned a great deal from that experience for my interrogation techniques when I interview clients in my bio-sig consultations. Nobody can lie to me: I will find out. I went through some life-threatening and mind-boggling fight or flight situations, and judging by the other guys who trained with me, it determines whether someone can deal with the extreme conditions and whether you can save a life by risking your own. However, being fit mentally and physically will always give you an edge, no matter what.

Here is what world–renowned coach **Charles R. Poliquin** has to say about this unique form of stress response: *"We are designed with an amazing physiological response to danger known as the 'fight or flight' response. If you were being chased by a saber-tooth tiger, your body would respond with a hormonal flood of adrenalin and cortisol, focusing all of your energy systems and attention towards surviving the encounter. For a short period of time, your body's priorities completely change from things like healing wounds, clearing toxins and digesting your breakfast to the much more immediate needs of survival. Just a few of the physiological reactions include: blood sugar skyrockets, heart rate and blood* *pressure increase, digestion slows, and even vision and hearing are altered. Everyone knows the signs and symptoms of an overt adrenalin rush, but problems arise when we are continuously in a low-grade fight or flight response."*

What does not kill you makes you **stronger,** so let me tell you that my intestinal fortitude got a lot stronger. I had the pleasure of attending a special course on close protection and security-related fields where all invited work to perfect their art. We went through every imaginable situation which could have gone wrong, and we never knew the outcome in advance. They just threw us in with a small briefing and let all hell break loose, and in some situations it did. It's a crazy world, and I got a taste of it.

Situation #1: We had to bring the VIP from Point A to Point B on a street intersection. Everything seemed normal, too normal. My partner had "the package", and I was about ten feet in front of them. Suddenly a nice tall blonde with a trench coat passed beside me (a decoy), but I didn't give a crap because I looked immediately at my partner and told him, watch your ass, it's going to blow some time soon. About ten seconds later, a guy came out of nowhere and started shooting at us. My partner shoved the VIP behind a barricade and so did I. Even though we were armed, I shot twice and so did the assailant. At least, that's what I heard.

After all was done, the teachers made us relive it, without the element of surprise. As we watched what happened, we learned that the assailant shot six times, while in the action I heard only two small pops, but when we relived it, the first shot was so loud that I didn't hear the five other gunshots. From that moment, I had mad respect for fight or flight. All my senses were focused on surviving and looking at who the hell was trying to kill us, so that's why I heard only two gunshots. We were doing the exercises inside a wide office space with some barricades and huge filing cabinets. As I dove to hide behind a cabinet, I made a huge hole in the wall, but didn't feel a thing, thanks to the adrenaline rush.

Situation #2: This is where I really got tested. We had to get out on the street, in a riot with a very important package. People had baseball bats and rocks, and they were screaming like crazy. As we got our foot out the door, a group of people came and charged at us. We had our guns drawn, pointing at the floor, but still they were aggressive and tried to get our package. As I was getting irritated, I yelled "STOP!" The fact that I yelled stop is not really surprising since we have to try and bring the tension down as much as possible before using other means. It's just how it came out. To me, it's as if I just yelled like that, but the power and loudness were surprising. Needless to say, the group was surprised, and everybody stopped. Even the instructors were shocked. For about five seconds, the silence was dense. That is when I said calmly, "Get the fuck out of the way, or I will go right through you." In martial arts we call it the KiAi, short exhalation before or during a strike or technique, used to startle and demoralize inexperienced or shy adversaries, so I guess mine worked relatively well.

I also had some hostage situations I had to deal with, covered mostly in my martial arts courses. Knowing how to calm down the situation was fundamental. Keeping your head cool and under control is what makes you successful, bringing down the tension before it degenerates. There is no room for heroes and Chuck Norris stuff in those fragile situations. However, I got to learn how to disarm and to take down someone, armed with a gun, knife or whatever he or she had, in a matter of seconds with quick reactions and joint locks (or breaks). My best experience was in getting myself out of a multiple assailant situation, with two people grabbing me by the arms and one holding me in a chokehold. It took me five seconds, and they were all on the floor in some kind of joint lock, and it worked every time, no matter how hard or what they grabbed. Grip training was the biggest influence in my martial arts training since judo and jiu-jitsu were the major elements in all the grabs and throw downs.

Where am I going with this? In life-threatening situations, the strong and healthy will prevail. I know people who, from the moment they feel stressed, see their digestion shut down, feel weak or just hide when the going gets tough. Some of us don't like to stay comfortable: we need constant brain stimulation and physical challenge. Make the comparison yourself. Look at most gym members, look for those who do cardio all the time while hardly changing their routines, and look at those who are thriving to lift heavier weights each time they work out and are pushing themselves harder at every session. Which one of these trainees shows the best results?

Those who push the envelope, those who want to get stronger, come out ahead, beyond a doubt. I saw a big difference in the courses between those who did cardio only because they thought it was important for their cardiovascular health and those who were getting their asses kicked in jiu-jitsu and grappling. Maybe I was a bit too hard on them to prove my point, but they understood. Those who thought they would have the edge in grappling because they could spend hours on a treadmill still got their butt kicked. You can't transfer an ability elsewhere. Running on a treadmill won't give you more endurance in grappling if you have no strength whatsoever. In my opinion, you train yourself to fight or to run away, thus the fight or flight stress response.

Define it however you want, in my book, I see it as intestinal fortitude. The will to push beyond your known limits, the strength to overcome fear, the mind-over-matter attitude. This is basic strength, your own. If you find the first little hidden strength that you can dig at, to overcome whatever goals you might have set yourself, the first few minutes of achievement will produce a sense of accomplishment and also that little adrenaline rush.

As you become stronger, you have that little rush more often. As you gain the strength to overcome fear, you have that little rush every time you do it. As you gain the strength to overcome obstacles and keep going, you have that little rush every time you do it.

Mental strength

In the next few weeks, as you start applying these new habits, you will soon understand that mental strength can be nourished. You can supply your brain with good habits and with the fuel it needs to function optimally. Let's start with the habit part. Strong-minded people have a lot of habits and qualities we can learn from. They are generally leaders and hard workers. They have strong opinions and beliefs.

Mental strength is not easy to obtain. It must be practiced everyday. It is like weightlifting. If you want to become stronger, you must lift every day. The same goes for mental strength: you need to keep your mind working to keep it strong. You need to feed it not only with the right nutrients but with the right thoughts and environment as well.

Whatever happened in the past, never feel sorry for it

Whatever happened has happened. Don't complain about your situation if it gets critical. Just keep your eyes on the prize. Understand fully that the present moment is the result of what you have worked for, good or bad.

When we found out that my friend had knee cancer, we obviously had to stop everything. Now, all that was important was my friend Stephen's treatment and recovery. We suddenly forgot everything we were preparing for, and all our attention was focused on the now, the present moment. But I must tell you that, whatever happened after the diagnosis, these were among the hardest moments of my life. Seeing a big man, who a few months earlier, even though he was limping and almost unable to stand on his leg due to constant pain, was able to fight three black belts in Seiza position (kneeling) and beat the crap out of us. He fought in the army, worked as a protection agent for the government and was brought to his knees by an unknown force.

The hardest time was when he had to get his leg amputated to stop the cancer from spreading (this was already too late since he already had some metastasis in his lungs). I remember his face as if it was just yesterday. I went to see him the next day, and I saw something in his eyes that I will never be able to put into words. I saw one of the strongest men I knew come down to his feet. I saw a powerful and fearless warrior who saw death eye-to-eye and ordered it to fuck off, admit he was defeated, and ready to give up. I saw someone whom I looked up to look up to me, and without talking, clearly asked for strength. In his mind, he lost his ability to fight, he lost all strength. While he endured so many life-threatening fights in the army, and protected a few high dignitaries and political figures, it never came to his mind that something so fierce could render him powerless without his consent, or at least without a fight.

There is an old saying that until you have been Ronin seven times, you can't become a real samurai. You must have seven falls and stand up eight times. A week or so later, he got up again. He fought the best he could and did his best to enjoy the time left with his awesome wife and two beautiful young girls. He died a year later, a real samurai.

> *"There is surely nothing other than the single purpose of the present moment. A man's whole life is a succession of moment after moment. There will be nothing else to do, and nothing else to pursue. Live being true to the single purpose of the moment."*
> — *Yamamoto Tsunetomo*

They seek control

Trying to control every aspect of your life is enough to make you go crazy. However, whatever aspect you CAN control, do so. Mastering important habits will help you gain control of your health and mental state. If these two aspects of your life are optimal, the rest will always come somewhat more easily.

They don't fear change

The problem with this is that the brain doesn't actually give a fuck about dreams or goals. So being constant is the key. Understand that you have some kind of control over your thoughts and some external influences. You can't let procrastination or easier and often meaningless tasks get in your way. Constantly practice the big-rocks-first principle. If a given task demands some major change, tackle it head on, without more than one thought. Change is good. Change is uncomfortable. Change challenges everything. If it doesn't change you, the challenge is not great enough. Change is good.

All or nothing

Know that some decision may lead to failure. Your desire for success should dominate your fear of failure. Once you have accepted the fact that failure is inevitable, but also a learning experience, giving your all seems like the only logical way, you win either way.

Total focus

If you can't control it, don't bother. Leaders don't even pay attention to things they can't control. If you need to pay attention to a problem that can be changed and worked on, do so, but never waste your time on stupidities.

Chapter 5

Get Stronger

Now that we have seen how to balance the mind, it is time to take care of the body. Unfortunately, this is a book, not a private coaching lesson. As you have read many times, individualized training is the key to success. The best I can do is to give you basic guidelines. However, I would still suggest that you consult a qualified trainer. Look for someone who has experience and who can show you results with past clients.

I'll be brief but to the point. I want to give you the best hints: for beginners, on how to start; for those with experience but stuck on a plateau, how to get better; and for old–timers, tips on how to make them last as long as possible.

You are a weightlifting newbie ...

1. Start with the basics. Don't try Ronnie Coleman's Olympia workout because you won't feel shit and you'll get destroyed. You need to wake up your metabolism and your mind-muscle

connection. Do three sets of 12 to 15 for each major muscle with a rest of 60 seconds between each set. For example:

A: flat barbell bench press, 3 sets of 12 with a minute between each set.
B: one-arm bent-over row, 3 x 12 with 60 seconds rest.
C: leg press, 3 x 15, with 60 seconds rest.
D: lying leg curl, 3 x10, with 60 seconds rest.
E: dips, 3 x 10, with 60 seconds rest.
F: standing barbell curl, 3 x 12, with 60 seconds rest.

Do this for six to eight weeks, and then you have two choices: hire a trainer to build you a program, or just read whatever you can, especially the next few pages by considering your training age (e.g., you have been training for three years, so your training age is exactly that).

2. You will gain lean muscle fast in the beginning, but only if you do what you have to. Eat protein, veggies and fats at every meal, which should be at least three to four times a day. Yes, everything you do will bring you results because your body craves it, but it will slow down. There will be adaptation. It's common among kids and beginners to see them gain a fair amount of lean mass in a few months.

3. It will not get easier. Since adaptation will be knocking on your door soon, you'll have to bust your ass a bit more,

assuming you get past the first year. Then again, most of you won't. Sad, but it is what it is. I don't know a lot of people who started training and kept it going for at least a year. All you have to do is prove me wrong.

4. Do your own shit. It doesn't matter what your pumped-up friends tell you, it doesn't mean you'll have the same results. You may try it, but keep in mind that you are not the exact copy of your friends, so what works for them may not work for you.

5. Respect experience. I am not talking about your pumped-up friends. Look for people who had results, not only with them but with other people or clients. This speaks volumes, and you'll probably **hear** the experience when you talk to them. Look for the no-bullshit approach.

6. Read as much as you can. When you start training, fitness magazines are good. Simple and short information is best. You will soon see that it can get very confusing. Try it out and take notes. It will be useful in the next few years.

7. What you do now has an impact on the rest of your life. Stamp that in your head – with a shovel.

8. You are probably looking for a quick fix, which does not exist and never will. You probably are looking for short cuts, which you will learn shortly. These can save you only a few work-outs due to possible injuries and overuse.

9. Please, no curls in the squat rack, unless you can curl what someone can squat.

You are an advanced trainee

10. You should have at least a year or two under your belt. If you're lucky, no injuries and a little muscle mass made its way onto your frame. You should also be thinking that you are plateauing, which you are not. You just may be lacking a new program or some new principles.

11. You kept on doing what you liked and started taking out what you disliked, which is a big mistake. Those huge lifts you are not doing are actually what you should be doing.

12. Don't forget the basic lifts like bench presses, dead lifts and squats.

13. I have to introduce to you a new friend, the pull-up. I know you saw some freak do it in the gym, but you should do it as well. It is one of the greatest upper body builders around. It's hard? You can bet your ass it is. I told you it would not get easier. At least it shouldn't.

14. If you had or have injuries, take care of them now. It will get worse.

15. You got a trainer! Well done. As long as he/she doesn't look at you doing cardio for 30 minutes, you should be fine.

16. Your readings should have evolved to fewer magazines, and to more experienced and specific publications. The Web is good, but it's easier to read contradictory views. Look for reputation, with results in numbers, and not only pictures of washboard abs, oiled-up arms or the number of likes they have on their Facebook page.

17. You may be considering getting certified. Good for you. Start with the basics again and learn from the best. The investment is well worth it. However, how you got in shape is not enough for coaching people. Get certified.

18. You still train two hours each session? Don't go past an hour from now on. Your adrenal glands will thank you for it. See your adrenals as energy reserves for the coming years.

19. The good thing is that you already figured out that it will always be a challenge. The fact that you kept this habit in your life for more than a few years speaks volumes. You know that it will never end, that you will always crave it and that it's a quest, not just a goal.

Old-timer weightlifters

20. You should still be on a quest.

21. You figured out almost everything you need to know about yourself, physically and, for the lucky ones, mentally. You

have learned how to deal with a lot of problems, physically and mentally.

22. Since you know a lot, you probably forgot a lot as well.

23. Even though you went back to the basics years ago, you seem to forget that you are not a 20-year-old any more. Fortunately, those who realize it don't give a shit about the new trends and the fresh little trainees with their personal best.

24. Understand that, if you have a bad workout, it was only that, a bad workout. On to the next one. Don't expect to recuperate the way you did in your younger years, even if you do everything right.

25. The best supplements in your case are still the basics, fish oils, multivitamins and some kind of joint support formula.

26. Never stop moving, and mostly do resistance training. The only thing that makes your bones strong is when you put pressure on them. The only way to do that is weightlifting and staying active. Calcium supplements and walking won't do shit.

27. Get to the gym for 30 minutes, four to five days a week. That's all you need. If you stop moving, you'll die slowly.

28. If you're a lucky one, you'll have no meds. If your doctor suggests that you take some, consider taking

charge and reverse these health concerns as soon as they come out. The only way to prevent it is to go for regular blood checks. No problems? Go maybe once a year. Have some concerns? Go run some tests now. Don't wait for it to be too late. Your body is a well-oiled machine, but you still need to give it a fighting chance. Do what you have to, eliminate what you know feeds the problems. and prove that living a healthy life goes a long way.

29. What's the point of saving money for retirement all your life if you can't take advantage of it when the time comes? Stay active as long as you can, and you'll be able to use your hard-earned money and take advantage of it with your loved ones.

30. Lead by example. Show the younger trainees how you did it. Maybe give some hints here and there. What I have learned is that the best ones will always go back and look at what was done before. They can learn from others' mistakes and realize the importance of experience. I personally keep an eye on new trends, but when I speak to someone of experience, I listen even more. I look at old-timers like an open book, and if I ask the right questions I get the right answers.

Last but not least, when it comes to health and fitness, tell people what they need to hear, not what they want to hear. It doesn't matter how conceited you may seem, and it doesn't matter that some people will be offended. What matters is that they will remember you when they have figured out that you were right.

These were more general guidelines, and how you should experience the way of life. When it comes to the actual workout, after a while, the body follows one rule, adaptation. When I say after a while, it means three to five weeks into your actual program. That is when it gets complicated and when a great trainer can keep the challenges coming. Now, as you gather experience, you need more variation. I want to expose you to some principles that I, as well as some of my fellow coaches, have used with great success with athletes, the regular Joes and on us. Some of the principles may sound like bro science and some are backed up by real science. Most if not all of them were the product of years under barbells that got mixed up and/or theories that got thrown away.

1. Volume

Whatever you are doing, do more, for a few weeks, three or four at most. Most guys get caught up in doing the prescribed number of sets for a given repetition scheme. That's fine, but after a while increase the volume (number of sets) by 40% for three weeks. So instead of doing six sets, do ten sets. Even if it doesn't make sense, do it. Shock the system once in a while.

2. Beta-alanine

Research has shown that using beta-alanine with creatine is the way to go. Beta-alanine increases carnosine, which increases power performance. Muscle carnosine is one of the more stable muscle metabolites because, once elevated, they are easily maintained and do not wash out once they are at maintenance levels. When supplementation is stopped, it may take as long as 20 weeks to wash out, compared to creatine, which washes out in less than four weeks.

Data suggest that β-alanine supplementation elicits a significant ergogenic effect when an exercise lasts one to four minutes. However, as with any studies, clear and precise testing, methodologies, supplement purity, the reliability of exercises for testing and measurement are required in future testing to produce and evaluate its efficiency.

3. Grip strength

The missing link in every guy's strength and endurance is grip strength. If your grip gets tired faster than the rest of the body, there's no way in hell you'll be able to improve work capacity in major muscle groups. Dead lifts, chin-ups, presses and trap bar squats are major body builders, but if you can't hold the bar, you are missing out. Your hand and fingers wrap ergonomically around the Gripsfear and improves your grip strength tremendously. Here is a little bonus, a little program for your grip strength and forearm thickness. Even your bones will feel pumped.

A1 wide pronated grip curl GripsFEAR x8 no rest

A2 medium pronated grip curls GripsFEAR x8

A3 close pronated grip curl x8 4 sets, 90sec rest between

B1 grips fear behind back wrist curls x12

B2 behind back wrist curls (no grips fear) AMRAP (same weight as B1) rest 30sec

B3 pronated wrist curl on bench bent elbow x8-10 (kneeling, forearms on bench, shoulders over elbows, no cheating allowed.) 4 sets, 90sec rest between

C1 supinated grip wrist curls 3xAMRAP (+-15) kneeling, forearms on bench, shoulders over elbows, no cheating allowed

"Who doesn't want superior strength and the ability to use more weight? But how often does your arm work stop at bis/tris, also known as Monday for the broscience community. When you have an imbalance of strength around a flexing & rotating joint like the elbow, injury becomes a question of when not if. One thing that will kill your gains faster than watching a Richard Simmons marathon is like having to rehab the elbow and take time off because the arm workout was halfway done. Strengthen and balance the musculature below the elbow with GripsFEAR and you will never be forced to choose which type of elliptical to use because of a bum elbow."

— Jared Leeper, GripsFear coach, owner, head Honcho, inventor

4. Angles

Instead of always doing the same angles such as the 30° inclined barbell bench press or the T-bar bench rows, I always advise my trainees to change the angle of attack. For example, the usual bench presses are always flat or inclined. When inclined, it is always the same 30° angle. So instead, I ask them to bring a single bench (commonly used for free weights) in the squat rack (as long as it is not for curls, you are allowed), and they have to put it at a 45° angle. As you will read in #12, it's always good to hit the chest at different angles, and new recruitment pattern for the shoulders as well.

5. Strength curves

Every exercise has a specific one, depending on body angles, injuries, trainee strength and experience, and equipment used. Simply put, an exercise that gets tougher at the end of the movement (end of concentric) has an ascending strength curve (pull-ups), an exercise that is easier at the end of the movement has a descending curve (bench press) and, finally, a concave strength curve is one that is hard at mid-point (standing barbell curls). By changing angles (#4), you change the strength curve.

My favorite way of changing the strength curve is to use gadgets like chains. If you use them on a barbell bench press for example, the weight on the bar gets heavier incrementally as you go up, which changes the strength curve from descending to ascending.

6. Zinc

Zinc plays a major role in anabolic hormone production. It is the key player in the production of the three most important muscle builders in the body, testosterone, growth hormone and IGF-1. It is also a major immune booster. Fewer sick days mean more gym days. Zinc also improves cell health. It builds enzymes necessary for insulin to bind to cells, which helps glucose to be used as fuel or stored as energy and helps build more lean muscle tissue, a.k.a. more gains.

7. Estrogen (take that shit out)

Estrogen impairs testosterone. Less testosterone = lower gains. More estrogen = fat gains. Not the gains we are looking for here. Estrogen, unfortunately, is omnipresent in our everyday life. Paraben in hand soaps, shampoos and perfumes are full of it. This is another sneaky kind of estrogen, a.k.a. xenoestrogen, an estrogen mimicker that has devastating effects on our bodies. Plastic bottles are a common transporter of xenoestrogen. A quick tip: never reheat your food in a microwave oven with plastic Tupperware. The plastic breaks down into micro particles and falls on your food. It also changes the molecular content of your food (no good), Just these two reasons are enough to reheat in a regular oven to get the most out of your meals.

8. Java stim

Designed to increase training drive without the usual crash of stimulants. On top of that, you get a dose of phenylalanine and tyrosine, which helps rebuild the adrenals, with all those hard workouts coming your way.

9. Multivitamins

It's a fact that what we eat these days is much lower in nutrients than what they had before. Adding a simple multivitamin to your daily meals can help tremendously. Let's say that you put cheap gas in your car: the engine will wear out faster, and anything attached to the engine will pay in the long run. The same goes for our bodies. Making sure you get the necessary supplements for detoxification and regeneration is the least you can do.

10. Supersets

There exist many kinds of supersets. In this case, to gain lean muscle mass, the first thing you can do is to superset two exercise for the same muscle group, one after the other with no rest between for maximum muscle damage. Remember, you don't grow in the gym, you rebuild outside of it. For example, here are some you could do for different muscle groups.

Chest: Flat bench press + dips (mechanical advantage)
Chest: High pulley crossover + flat bench press (pre exhaustion)
Quads: Sissy squats + barbell back squats (mech adv/pre exhaustion)
Quads: leg extension + leg press (pre exhaustion)
Posterior chain: barbell dead lift + penta jump (contrast training)
Biceps: Scott curl + supinated grip pull-ups (pre exhaustion)

11. Giant sets

This will get you to Swolebraham Lincoln levels fast. Same as 10, but just put it four or five exercises in a row. However, just don't pick any exercise out of your head. The best bet is to start with the hardest ones first and finish off with the easiest. When I say hardest, I mean the most neurologically challenging, like multi-joint exercises (dead lifts, squats, bench or chins) and finish off with machines. It would look like the following:

A1 Barbell front squats x8 no rest
A2 Barbell hack squats x10 no rest
A3 Leg press x15 no rest
A4 Leg extension x20 rest 120 seconds,
Repeat for 5 sets.

12. Mechanical advantage

Still seen as a superset, but with the same exercises used with different angles or grips. For example, the inclined bench press is tougher on an incline than on a decline (well, for most of us). So you basically start with the toughest version of an exercise and finish off with the easiest again, as per #11, except that since it is the same exercise, muscle fatigue is localized and comes much faster. So you could do a 60° press, followed by a 45°, than a 30°, 15°, flat bench and if you really are masochistic, finish it all with a 15° declined press. I forgot to mention that these are all done without rest in between, so from A1 to A6 there is no rest. Another way to do it would be on pull-ups.

A1 Wide pronated grip pull ups AMRAP no rest (As Many Reps As Possible)

A2 Close pronated grip pull ups AMRAP no rest

A3 Wide supinated grip pull ups AMRAP no rest

A4 Close supinated grip pull ups AMRAP no rest (by now, those are also called kipping pull-ups popularized by Crossfit)

A5 close neutral grip pull ups AMRAP rest 150 seconds and repeat for 4 sets

13. Strength

One of the major mistakes I see with those who want to gain muscle mass is that they focus too much on hypertrophy. They stick predominantly with a slow twitch and the IIa fast twitch fibers, which use a mixture of aerobic and anaerobic metabolism. What they should be doing is to periodize properly and include the IIa fast twitch fibers, predominantly for strength and power. Although getting stronger does not necessarily mean being strong, increasing your strength on the lower rep range spectrum will make you stronger for the higher six to 12 reps required to build muscle mass. The notion of time under tension becomes important in this case since it can increase gains tremendously, and manipulating them periodically helps bring results that last. More on the subject of tempo in #34.

14. Patient lifter

Enter German volume training. Usually, most will do a set of warm-ups and than jump right at max weight. On good days, they probably get to four good sets, but with only one or two at or near the chosen maximum rep range. With German volume, there are two possible ways to execute this workout. Keep the same weight and achieve all ten sets of ten repetitions at around 65% to 70% of your 1 RM, and increase the weight by 5% every workout, or use 75% of your 1 RM, and try to see how many sets you are able to hold at 10 reps. In this one, you will probably drop reps at about 5 sets, from ten to eight and then maybe seven repetitions. If you can't do more than six, decrease the weight by 5%, and so on. Once you have reached the critical drop-off point of 40% off the bar, you are done. That's the goal, to find your drop-off, and then to beat it the following workout. You should do better on the next workout.

15. Weakness

A chain is as strong as its weakest link. We all know what it is, and find it is boring to work on. However, if you put your full attention on it, it can be turned into your best weapon to improve all your other lifts. The best way to improve a weak spot or a "procrastinating" body part is to work on it twice a week. If you want to do even better, try it twice a week, twice a day or, if possible, every day, while alternating low reps on one workout and higher reps on the other. Morning basic lifts and higher volume (sets) of work, and night is focused on hypertrophy.

My favorite way to improve a weak part is to take two sessions a week, not counting sets but going for time instead. I dedicate 50 minutes of my day to these two body parts or exercises that I suck at. I did front squats and pull-ups in a superset style for 45 minutes, twice a week. I went from eight pull-ups to 15 (no kipping shit), and I increased my front squats by almost 65 pounds in a few weeks.

16. Back to basics

Never underestimate the power of going back to basics. Basic exercises, programming, simple tempo – just keeping it simple. It also has to be fun, more so after training for so many years.

17. Insulin sensitivity

As with #7 and zinc, insulin sensitivity is über important for overall wellbeing. Insulin sensitivity is the same as how well your car is tuned to use the fuel when you push the pedal to the metal. The better you take care of it, the better it will perform, exactly how it should be with our bodies. With most people I see coming in my office, more and more are insulin-resistant, which is the complete opposite. Not all carbohydrates are created equal, and some of them have a devastating effect on the body, short term and long term. Choose your food wisely because the saying is absolutely true, you are what you eat. One last thing: you don't have to live low-carb, you just have to choose them properly. I see carbs the same as my workouts, I like to cycle between high-carb periods and low-carb periods, depending on the goal and training protocols.

18. Cut carbs

I like to cut carbs when people come to see me for the first time. I like to cut carbs to shock the system into using stored fat as a source of energy. However, when you take something out of the diet, put something in. When you cut carbs, you increase fat intake. I cut carbs in bodybuilding protocols. But everything I just mentioned previously leads me to my next tip.

19. Add carbs

Once I have cut carbohydrates, I will ALWAYS try to reincorporate them slowly into the diet. I will use post-workout carbs in high-intensity protocols, even throughout the day. If you haven't understood this yet, A DIET PROTOCOL SHOULD BE INDIVIDUALIZED. There are no secret protocols, only baseline, which you work around once you do your homework. It takes way more than a bit of research or a few successful clients to understand someone's body. You may come across a great protocol, but that doesn't mean it will work the second time around. Trial and error will always be the game. Anyone who says otherwise is a fucking crook, in my opinion.

20. Up your protein intake

This debate has been going for many years, with results on both sides of the spectrum, high protein or the required minimum to gain lean mass. However, if you look at ALL the research available, we can conclude that those who took more than 1.5 grams per pound of bodyweight always gained more muscle mass. Although I am not a big fan of weighing food and calorie counting, my advice would be, whatever amount of protein you are eating now, eat more, and if you want to make sure, double that. I know, you can't keep eating huge amounts of meat all the time, and you are right! Like everything we do in weight lifting, cycle your protein intake. Alternate between high- and low-protein intake periods.

21. Add branched chain amino acids

They support liver health and detoxification, prevent diabetes and are über important for longevity, but the most important aspect of branched chain amino acids is their ability to help recovery and regeneration, to help users stay lean and strong, and to help improve work capacity.

They are a must.

22. Slack off the heavy sets

If you abuse strength training, your body and joints may suffer. I am talking about those who have the bodybuilding mindset but who always try to do their one-rep max on the bench every time they set foot in the gym. If it is periodized in your program, I am fine with that, but variety is the key. If you do so for long periods of time, you will even see your max on the bench go down. Your joints will pay the price, and if you use strength protocols for extended periods of time, more than a few months consecutively without rest or de-loads (dropping the number of sets by 40%), you may be on your way to overtraining, and even adrenal fatigue. This leads me to my next tip.

23. Periodization

When we talk about periodization, we often think of Olympics and athletes. In a way, bodybuilders are athletes and should at least use a very simple form of periodization, called "change." Guys (and gals), I know how much you like to train your arms or chest, but it's a matter of balance. Hypertrophy needs to be alternated with periods of strength and vice versa. The body adapts very quickly to a given rep range, and we all know that hypertrophy is mostly from 6 to 12 repetitions. As discussed in point #13, dig into the IIb fibers for three to four weeks for time under tension below 20 seconds per set, than go back up to between 40 and 70 seconds per set, and as a bonus finish off with back-off sets of 20 reps or TUT of more than 70 seconds with the last exercise of the day. If you change your programs often, faster results will be the outcome.

24. Post-workout shakes

Don't underestimate the power of a post-workout shake. Protein synthesis and muscle growth are optimized when protein is consumed immediately after a workout. For even better results, add glycine, which lowers cortisol (a big no-no after a workout) and glutamine, which helps restore muscle glycogen levels and accelerates recovery after a workout.

25. Post-workout nutrients

I would highly suggest Vitamin C for everyone, especially for those with adrenal issues. A 2008 study had untrained men take one gram of vitamin C pre-workout and do 30 minutes of moderate exercise. Post-workout cortisol levels dropped more rapidly than a placebo group, and the effect was apparent directly after exercise, and at two and 24 hours post-workout. I also recommend magnesium – serious trainees are depleted. It speeds up recovery from strenuous training, helps regenerate the adrenals and also lowers cortisol.

26. Water

Most people train in almost dehydrated states. Did you know that a decline of as little as 1% in water could result in a 10% strength loss? So drink a boatload of water. There are formulas out there. But let's keep it simple: the more active you are, the more you need. Gals should drink at least two to three liters a day and guys four to five liters, if not more.

27. Booster drinks

Of the numerous problems with energy drinks, the worst one is well hidden. The medical and fitness community are interested these days in natural and man-made toxins called <u>obesogens</u>. Those endocrine disruptors are found in very common products, such as corn syrup, and chances are that if you are a big fan of energy drinks, you have some endocrine disrupting going on. The other problem is the hidden sugar. They are comparable to soft drinks, even the sugar-free ones.

If you need energy in a can, don't look at a can for the solution, look at what is causing you to look for a can as a solution.

But there is more…

28. Mind games

Another problem I find with those drinks is that it gives you wings (Red Bull line), but what happens when you run out? You fall on your face. It gets to be a psychological game. When you try to stop or you can't have one on a given training day, you think you absolutely need it for a good workout. You think you can't train the same, so you just go easy or just don't train at all.

29. Sleep

As you have read in the 12 habits, it's all a matter of quality. If you can't sleep a full night without waking up, then you may want to look into it. However, sleeping for more than eight hours a night may also be a problem. Sometimes more is not better. Every time I ask the question "are you sleeping well?" most people say they are. Beauty is in the eye of the beholder. Great sleep means different things to different people.

The problem is that there is many ways in which you can easily disturb your sleep. To keep it simple, here are some simple tips if you have a hard time sleeping or getting sleepy:

1. Dim the lights an hour before bedtime.
2. Don't watch anything that could excite or stress you – action flix, porn (obviously), news or anything that could fire you up.
3. Have a pre-bed routine.
4. Read a book.
5. Under no circumstance should you use a computer, Kindle, IPad or phone less than an hour before bedtime.

Yes, it's boring. But if you don't sleep, you don't regenerate, and you impair night-time growth hormone production. These are two of the main mechanisms that will help in your quest for muscular gains.

30. Multiple workouts a day

If you have the luxury of having time for two or even three short workouts a day, I would strongly urge you to do it. You don't have to do it for months, just a few short weeks, to boost results through the roof. Here are some possible permutations:

AM: high volume (sets), low reps;
PM: hypertrophy-based workouts (supersets, giant sets);
or
AM: power, Olympic lifts, strongman;
PM: strength training;
or
AM: energy systems;
PM: hypertrophy training, fat loss weight training circuits.

For daily multiple training sessions, use shorter sessions (40 minutes max), which are more efficient. More importantly, choose the most-bang-for-your-bucks exercises. For fast gains, same body parts twice a day are suggested.

31. De-load

Training four, five, eight, ten or 15 sessions a week, you have to de-load, at least every 12 weeks. Each program should last about four weeks. On the third week, bring down the volume by 40%. It is not a because it is called a "de-load" week that you have to take it easy: go all out, but for fewer sets, six sets instead of ten, for example.

32. Boost your brain the natural way

The meat and nuts breakfast (habit #1) is the best natural way to do it. What you eat for breakfast sets up your neurotransmitters for the day. Dopamine helps with energy, interest, and motivation. Acetylcholine controls mental acuity and memory. The production of acetylcholine is inherently dependent on dietary fat and choline.

33. Functional hypertrophy

The problem with most guys in gyms is that they become lazy. We all want to get big and strong, but lifting heavier every session creates strain or is just plain dangerous. Functional hypertrophy is just another way of doing supersets, except that it is, in my opinion, the better way to get big. Heavier and eccentrically more challenging, it gets you strong AND big at the same time, hence "functional" hypertrophy. For example, a simple leg workout would look like this:

A1 Barbell front squats 5 reps 60x0 10 sec rest.
A2 Trap bar squats 5 reps 60x0 60 sec rest
A3 Lying leg curl 5 reps 60x0 120 sec. rest
Repeat A1 to A3 for 5 sets.

34. Varying tempo

For those not familiar with tempo, 60×0 would mean lowering the weight in six seconds, with no stop (0) at the bottom, X means to explode back up, (0) means no pause at the top, and so on.

Incorporating tempo into your workouts will only help you respect your hypertrophy protocol. To achieve hypertrophy, the time under tension (working set) would have to be between 40 and 70 seconds. So if you don't care about tempo and just go at it for eight to ten reps, which is what bodybuilders do, without slowing it down, you could have a time under tension of 20 to 25 seconds, which is more on the strength spectrum than on hypertrophy.

10 reps at a 1-0-1-0 tempo comes out to: 20 second time under tension.
10 reps at a 3-0-2-0 tempo comes out to: 50 seconds TUT.
The choice is obvious.
Control your tempo.

35. Negative

Finish off with a rep or two of negatives/eccentric lowering. Once you have fatigued the concentric part, which should be around your last good rep, lower the weight for ten seconds, twice or three times, until you can't hold the weight any more. If you can do more than 3 negatives, it was not heavy enough. You obviously need a spotter for those last repetitions. Maximum muscle damage produces greater hypertrophy. The eccentric part is the most efficient part of the lifts, by the way. This is another reason for using tempo.

36. Training like athletes

What I like to do to break beat is to use contrast training, as I do with my athletes. What is the use of training if you can't at least transfer these abilities outside the gym, like jumping, lifting fast or just trying to lift heavy shit once and putting them down. Simply put, some slow and controlled lifting followed by power and/ or explosive shit. Here are some examples:

Deadlifts + heavy bag throw down
Barbell squats + prowler AFAP 20 meters push
Trap bar dead lifts + penta jump
Five sets of five of these bad boys will leave you changed. You dig deep to recruit more fibers to execute the plyo or power moves.

37. Strongman

In the same vein, why not try some strongman. Lifting heavy tires, handling stones or just pulling and pushing heavy sleds and prowler digs in your intestinal fortitude. You like to feel the pump? I have never heard about anybody who pushed a prowler for 50 meters for a couple of sets who didn't have a hard time walking afterwards due to the huge pump in the quads.

Here is an example of a "modified strongman" workout.

A tire flips 6x6 rest 120 seconds between sets
B farmers walk 5x 50 meters rest 120 sec between sets
C heavy prowler push high handles 4x20 meters rest 90 seconds between sets

Due to the heavy demands on the nervous system, strongman style workouts are suggested once or twice a week only.

38. Change it up

For all the obvious reasons in the few last tips you have read, changing things around can only make you better. The best program is the one you are not doing. It takes a few weeks for your body to adapt to a given program, and the more experience you have, the faster you'll need the change. If it doesn't challenge you, it doesn't change you. Don't get comfortable, ever.

39. Eat more calories than you burn

For the calorie freaks, eat more than you can burn. Determine your caloric needs, and make sure to top that and then some. I do believe in feeding what the body needs and recognize. What he is able to breakdown and use as energy or to regenerate and find homeostasis. I don't really believe in counting calories, but if it makes you feel like a better person, go ahead. Just remember that a thousand calories of chips does not have the same impact on your body than a thousand calories of vegetables.

40. Go for the feel

I'm all for the go-heavy-or-go-home mentality, but the biggest problem when you always try to go heavy is that you don't actually feel what you're working. That is reason #236 why tempo is important. Moving a given weight in a controlled fashion, focusing on the absolute best contraction possible of the targeted muscle group, can only help in achieving the very important mind-muscle connection.

41. And for the pump

Supersets are great and functional hypertrophy is even better, in my opinion. But one of the best way to #feelthepump is the pre-fatigue/exhaustion principle. Use a concentration exercise in high reps to pre-fatigue a specific muscle and then use a multi-joint exercise that targets the same muscle as a prime mover.

High pulley crossovers + bench presses
Leg extensions + barbell back squats
Leg curls + stiff-legged dead lifts
Scott curls + standing barbell curls

However, here are two of the most important facts about that coveted pump feeling.

First, learn when to stop. That great handicapped like feeling that you can't move or that it will soon explode can be gone on the next set. Doing another set can be the difference between a huge crazy arm busting pump and a deflated balloon.

Second, although it's nice to get a pump every single workout, it will not always happen that way. It could be a matter of a few bad habits like lack of sleep, diet problems, hydration or just plain training adaptation that settled in.

42. Change your program often

Often means every four to six weeks as a rule of thumb. The older you are in training age, the faster you should change them. The more advanced you are in the gym, the faster you adapt to a certain type of training. So if you want to keep the results coming, change them once adaptation starts settling in.

43. Know your fat, then lose some

Want to look more muscular? Lose fat. If all you want to do is get bigger, fine. Although carrying fat may make you look bigger, it may slow you down a bit. That's just excess weight, dead weight. If you do your job well, gaining muscle and losing fat at the same time is possible and not that hard to do.

44. Planned overtraining

This is where it gets interesting. Without going into technical details, a bit of overtraining cannot do any harm if done properly. However, you may want to jump straight to #50 for this one. No one is the same, and if you don't plan it properly, you may jeopardize your health and your results in the long run.

It is hard to quantify just because of the fact that no one is the same. However, two to three weeks of pushing over the limit can just make those re-feeds very beneficial. I do that when some of my clients and athletes go on vacation. I know what they can or can't tolerate. So three to four weeks before they go away, I push them extra hard by increasing volume or adding some energy system training sessions to their programs. The fact that they will eat shit on vacation will just help them recuperate and won't mess up my plan, their plan.

45. Planning re-feeds

You have to earn your carbohydrates and cheat meals. Although we know a lot more people who can't go without their carbs than people who can live without them, I truly believe that we all need to re-feed once in a while. It's a question of motivation. Deprive yourself of a simple pleasure, and it isn't fun anymore. Did you know that you could be motivationally depleted? Yep, you can actually be out of motivation. I don't like to tell people that they have earned their right to eat a cookie – it just looks like I am rewarding a dog. I see it as planned re-feeds, to help our minds and body relax and enjoy what has been done, to show why we can actually enjoy eating what we like once in a while, but always without overdoing it.

46. De-stress

Very simply, stress = cortisol = catabolic. Catabolic = losing muscle mass. Taking stress out of your life, energy drainers, wankers. Sleeping when you can, even a nap during the day, which is a luxury for most of us, can have a great impact on your results. Just live one day at a time, train, and make time for stuff or people you enjoy, who makes you a better person. Have fun, and just enjoy every single minute of your life.

47. Energy systems

The most underestimated and underused system of them all. I am not talking about the cutting phase of bodybuilders who go on treadmills a few months before a show or beach season. I am talking about intervals, cardio capacity. It helps bring out vascularity, which helps the blood flow to the muscles, which helps get bigger muscles. It's science bro, bro' science.

48. Dropping the cardio

Am I contradicting myself with this? NO! I am talking about steady boring pace cardio. If you didn't get it by now, to trick your body into building lean muscle mass, you have to challenge it. The same goes for the cardio. Think about it, if you have a better cardiovascular capacity and can endure harder and longer workouts, the gains are yours. Focus on short intervals twice a week. Here is what I give to some of clients.

Team Prowler, three sets of 50 meters (I go, you go), rest two minutes, repeat three to four times; heeelllooo puke bucket).

Jacobs ladder, six to ten intervals of one minute work, one minute off.

Front squats ten seconds work, 20 seconds rest, for eight sets. Repeat two to three times. If you don't feel your quads with this, you never will.

49. Magnesium

I don't know if it's possible to keep it simple or short in explaining what magnesium can do to help us with our muscle gains. It's easier for me to say what it doesn't. Anyway, people who train regularly are almost always depleted in magnesium. You basically need magnesium for muscle contractions, for ATP, for energy. If you want to make sure you have adequate levels, get your red blood cell magnesium checked.

50. Investing

How can you know if you have gained lean muscle mass? How can you fix a goal if you don't actually know how much lean muscle mass you have at the moment or how much fat you need to lose? Exactly. Get yourself tested by a trainer or coach, and ask questions. Invest in a thorough evaluation, a few programs with a professional and at least, you won't have to look back at what went wrong with a big question mark on your forehead. Some of these tips are easily applicable, but others may be a little tricky if not done properly. Invest in yourself and guarantee some results.

Good to go? Wait. Now that you know what to do, it's always good to have a little list of what NOT to do as a reminder. Here is a little "most common" mistakes list that can help you avoid some setbacks, and a few reasons why.

Warming up or lack of

A warm-up should be thought of as a movement that will prepare your joints prior to heavier loads. So it should be specific with lighter weights than you would use for the first set of your exercise. Let's say you're doing squats: you can start by doing a regular squat with the empty bar, but don't do more reps than what you do in your actual workout. Then use maybe 50% of your working weight, again never doing more reps than intended in your workout. Doing more reps will set up your muscle into doing more reps and will break the intended effect. Doing warm-up sets of 20 repetitions when your repetition range should be six will send out faulty messages to your muscles.

Lifting too heavy

Lifting to impress your friends is a major mistake. You could pay with an injury for a long time. The only one you should impress is yourself. Who gives a crap if you can do three plates on the bench? As long as you push more than the last workout, that should be your goal. Then there are those who, when they increase, boost their total weight by ten pounds (five pounds on each side), if not double. The 2½-pound weights exist for a reason, for small increments, and if you are man enough, you will increase by even less. Let's say you have five reps to do with 300 pounds. You worked up slowly to 300 and are able to do two sets with 300 pounds. So instead of increasing by five pounds on each side, which brings you to 310 but with reps lowered perhaps to three or four, increase by one or 1½ pounfd. How? There are the micro-increment Pace weights available that can even increase your total weight by ½ or ¾ of a pound. Let me show you in total training volume. Numbers tell the true story. Let's say your goal is to complete 300 pounds for five sets of five repetitions.

Sets	Accident-waiting-to-happen way	Slowly-but-surely way	Goal
1	5x300	5x300	300
2	5x300	5x301.5	300
3	3x310	4x303	300
4	2x320	4x304	300
5	2x315	4x305	300
Total volume	5,200 lbs.	6,655.5 lbs.	7,500 lbs.

It's pretty obvious that "slowly-but-surely" is the way to go. Small increments at every workout are much more productive. This is just an example, but it is something that you can apply to every exercise, especially on small muscle groups such as the rotator cuffs, where an increase of only five pounds is most often impossible. If you don't have access to the Pace weights or plate mates, you could use barbell clips. They usually weigh about half a pound each. Just put one or two clips on each side to increase the total weight by one or two pounds. This is simple, and it does the job.

Lifting too light

This one is for the ladies, or those who are scared of getting too big too fast. Gain one pound of lean mass, burn 50 calories more a day. Gain ten pounds, burn off 500 calories a day doing what? Nothing!!! You just speed up your metabolism by doing so. You think gaining ten pounds of lean mass will make you look like a freak? It will only show as new shapely definition. Do you think a lady would look like a freak with ten pounds more on her frame? It will only show as more definition and less fat. It happens automatically because of the increased metabolism boost you get from your newly acquired lean muscle mass. Anyhow, an increase in lean mass never comes without a decrease in body fat. Higher buttocks, smaller hips, nicely defined arms, increased energy, solid workouts – but woman don't care, as long as the weight comes down (do you sense the sarcasm?).

Same exercises, day in, day out

People are always doing what they feel most comfortable doing. It's easier, and you look stronger since you have mastered the exercise for so long, but what if I tell you that, if you leave it for a couple of weeks or even months, focusing on your weaknesses, you would get stronger on that particular lift? The best example is the bench press. You see big boys going on the bench press as soon as they come in, put a plate of 45 pounds on each side and crank up a dozen of reps as fast as if they were using a shake weight. If someone wants to increase their bench, the first thing I do is get them off of it. I would focus on the scapular chain, pull-ups, and of courses some kind of pressing exercise, anything that would not involve a flat plane, instead using inclines and shoulder presses, chains and fat grips.

Full range, yeah right...

It really bothers me when I see someone on the bench or the squats that does not use full range, even more so when a trainer is suggesting it. If your joints bend all the way, maybe it is because it was meant to be. Always use a full range to lessen your chances of injury. Yes, you read that correctly, to LESSEN your chances of injury. How many times do I hear guys telling me that they cannot squat all the way down and that's why they go only half-way? What you create is a faulty biomechanical pattern that will overuse one part of the strength curve. Maybe your trainer prescribed it for specific reasons, which is quite possible. If it's because you think you are injured, or actually are injured, fix the problem first, or it will only make matters worse.

Too much cardio

Cardio should be case-specific. In other words, if you are training for a marathon, do long, steady-pace cardiovascular workouts to improve your time. If your goal were to compete in a 100-meter sprint competition, then doing cardio endurance (marathon) would impair your results. What you need is to work on cardiovascular power and also strength training to help you get faster.

If it is for **fat-burning** purposes, there are many schools of thought on the subject. I like to use sprints and interval training (short bursts of high-intensity work like rowing or sprinting followed by rest periods equal to working time) twice a week. A good nutritional plan and interval should get you lean in about six to eight weeks. Some like to use long steady-pace cardio sessions to get lean, especially those who are participating in physique contests. It works for some, and doesn't for others. Trial and error is always the name of the game. Please, don't go by the eye. It cracks me up when I see coaches look at their clients and say that they got leaner. That's just second-guessing your results and the hard work you have put into achieving them. Most coaches are scared of taking actual body fat measurements for fear of seeing no results or an actual increase in the body fat percentage. Be honest with yourself. A new training plan should start with a new body fat reassessment. It is the only way to know whether it worked or not.

Training too much

Sometimes less is more. Depending on your schedule, your lifestyle or your goals, I have one principle that is a very basic one, balance. Train like a madman and eat like a bird, I give you a couple of weeks and over-training is going to knock on your door. So put all your effort into all the elements, which are nutrition, a healthy and realistic lifestyle and the proper training for your needs, and you will reach your goals quickly.

Train or get out

So much time is wasted in gyms it's ridiculous. Depending on the gym where you signed up, you may have a geriatric population to deal with, which may be frustrating at times. Chances are you won't see them on the squat rack, but on the easier machines. However, some old-timers may be going at it harder than you. Use your gym time as "me time." Leave your phone in the locker, set small talk aside and use every single minute for a purpose. It will be used for work or for rest.

Chapter 6

Feeding The Warrior

I can tell you know this will be the shortest chapter. First things first: most of us have developed a bad relationship with food. We eat for comfort, reward, pleasure and to practice mathematics (bad bad calorie counting...). The only way to fix that is by adding another habit we did not talk about yet.

> *"Let food be thy medicine and medicine be thy food"*
> — *Hippocrates*

David Blaine, the street magician, likes to do simple card tricks but also loves to push the human performance. He was buried alive in a clear box underneath three tons of water for seven days. Blaine also performed a 72-hour stunt where one million volts of electricity was sent through his body, with the whole thing live-streamed over YouTube. He recently gave a Ted talk (go see it, I think it is one of the best) on how he managed to hold his breath for more than 17 minutes. He tried to figure out all the possible strategies on how he could beat the previous record of eight minutes and 58 seconds set by Tom Setias. To succeed in this challenge, he had to lose weight. He was 6 foot 1 and 250 pounds. Fat and big–boned, as he put it. The goal was to drop 50 pounds in three months. *What he ate in the next few months was seen as medicine.* Anything he had to eat was exactly what his body needed as nutrients to help him lose weight and recover from his extensive training.

Everything he ate had a purpose and was considered medicinal for the body, which is how we should see our daily nutritional intake. We should not eat for taste or until we feel full, but to satisfy a need. Not the need to calm cravings but to feed our body with the fuel it needs to perform optimally every single day. I know there are so many diets out there that it can be confusing. In my opinion, the Paleo and Mediterranean diets are those I've seen people get the best results from. However, Paleo is basically centered on what our ancestors ate, meat, veggies and fats. I'm fine with that, but I don't recall reading anything about *Paleo cheesecake* in evolutionary research. So stick with the basics. Every meal should have a portion of protein/meat (anything that was alive before), three to four portions (about 2-3 cups) of colored veggies (peppers, cauliflower, tomatoes, broccoli, sweet potatoes, etc.) and a portion (1-2 tablespoon) or two of healthy fats (avocado, nuts, oils, butter, etc.). Fruits? Sure, but one a day or just once in a while. I know fruits are supposed to be good for you, but as with anything else, do not abuse them. If overeaten, fruits could, in the long run, have the same response as a small chocolate bar. I won't go into details, as there is plenty of information out there. May I repeat again, **keep it simple.**

How many calories? Think of eating until you are satisfied but not full, never full. Gals should eat three to four meals a day and guys four to five. What about snacks? The problem I have seen with snacks is that they can disturb your appetite in many ways. Little snacks treats are just that, often full of sugar. Unless you are willing to have a healthy snack like veggies and a small portion of protein, I don't even see the use of calling them snacks, which is why I rather call them small meals. I usually take out the notion of snacks and implement the notion of four equally portioned meals. Due to the complicated nature of diets and individual nutritional requirements, I highly suggest you do a little research on this, or go and consult a certified trainer / fat loss / hypertrophy expert. This is money well invested for long-term results.

How much protein in a meal? As much as you are willing to eat. The usual rule is as big and thick as the palm of your hand.

Shouldn't you cut down on calories if you want to lose weight? I have seen so many different cases with different outcomes. For example, I had one girl who was eating two meals a day, on a good day. She always complained of feeling bloated and gained weight. I gave her four equally portioned meals a day with protein, veggies and healthy fats, and she started to lose weight and became a different woman in a matter of weeks. For some, I have to cut calories but not by going Hitler–calculated, as some trainers would do. I play with foods. Let's say someone ate baked potatoes and rice often, I would try to change that for wild rice and sweet potatoes. Fewer high glycemic index calories means a better insulin response.

Instead of bananas or apples, I switch them to berries for the same reasons.

How much water should I drink in a day? More than you are doing now. Active women should be near the two-to-three-liter mark, and guys should be closer to four to five liters a day. I know this seems like a lot, but it is one of the most underestimated elements of anyone's diet.

Isn't fat the enemy? Absolutely not. Since people started cutting fat from their diets, especially in the 1980s, obesity has been skyrocketing. A little fat at every meal will go a long way. To eat fat is to lose fat.

On the question of supplements, I rarely use them at first. If you don't do the basics like eating small but frequent meals, chewing your food properly to improve your digestion and working on the code of major habits, most supplements won't work. You may consider getting the basics such as a good multivitamin and fish oils since they can help in many ways when you start a new lifestyle change. Fish oils can help decrease inflammations and insulin sensitivity, and they increase serotonin levels, helping decrease the incidence of depression, anxiety, panic attacks and carbohydrate cravings. Besides that, I would start by doing everything right and then revise your complete protocol. For supplements, I would advise you to consult with a Poliquin-certified Bio-Signature practitioner near you. They can individualize your supplement protocol according to your specific needs. This will make you save a ton of money on useless supplements that most often, in terms of quality, won't do a thing for your goals.

Why do we need supplements? The food we eat is much lower in nutrients than before due to mass production and all the pesticides and antibiotics involved. We in turn have evolved and adapted around epigenetics. The environment has slowly modified our ancestors' DNA to the point that it changes each generation's genetic markers. For instance, we find ourselves more and more lacking vitamin D and magnesium, not only because stress and our digestion of processed foods makes it harder to get adequate levels of essential nutrients but also because our cells are not recognizing these nutrients as much as they should, with signals being smoked. Chemicals in our environment play a big role in how our cells absorb these nutrients and affect their function. Our bodies are exposed to at least 50 chemicals, and that's before 9 o'clock in the morning. The chlorine in the shower, the Parabens in creams and soaps, the coffee preservatives, the morning cigarettes, the cars on our way to work all have an effect.

> "What we do in life echoes in eternity"
> — Maximus

Our goal should be to control as best we can our environment, not the grass or water, but what we feed our body with, where we live, what we put our body through, the creams, scents and stress that put a toll on our system, affecting our genes. What we do now not only has a great impact on the rest of our lives but also on future generations, what science refers to as epigenetics.

Believe it or not, by eating right, you can help improve your genes and those of your kids before they set foot in this world. For many years people thought, and still do, that we are stuck with the body we have and that you can't reverse genes, but prevention and eating lean is what we need to focus on. If you want to live a healthy life and have great longevity, you must have great habits and stay active. Movement is life. As soon as you stop moving, the body ages.

Chapter 7

Let's Get To It

> "God gave us the gift of life; it is up to us to give ourselves the gift of living well."
> — Voltaire

You probably just put the book down and already have second thoughts. It's normal. This is a big step. You just understood the fact that it is not a diet or a new fad. All that you just have read is what everyone should do. Warriors or not, we need to take care of our bodies and treat them as temples. Most people do not have the luxury of having breads or little bowls of cereals at their convenience, every single day. Close protection officers eat what they have when they can. Olden warriors were the same. They actually stuck with the same foods. Trying different foods was a risk. They didn't know if they could digest new foods very well or if they would feel good after their meals. At time of war in particular. gluttony was out of the question, since it could impair or lessen their ability to fight. This sounds a bit extreme, if you ask me, but in olden days it may have meant life or death. Nowadays, it is a question of choice and availability.

I really don't want you to finish this book and do as you did with some previous books you may have read. I want you to start applying now only one of the code's 12 habits. Don't think about the diets or the training programs yet. Let's start by conquering a little fear. For example, you can't figure out how you can get to eat in the morning. Most people in your shoes simply don't have the time. My question to you is: why be like everyone else? Why would you want to be like them? Prove their theory wrong.

Another example could be that you always have to bring work home and do it once the kids are in bed. Fine, just set tasks and times to achieve them. If you want to go to bed at a given time like 11 p.m., do the most you can up until 9:30 or 10 p.m. Then, wake up early and finish the work while having your coffee and your meat and nuts breakfast. This way, you can fix three habits at once. First, prioritizing the big rocks, second, having a decent bedtime, and third and last, eating a great breakfast in the morning while working with a fresh and rested mind.

Find the one habit that can help a few at the same time. Some people eat before going to bed but complain they can't lose weight and/or can't eat breakfast in the morning. It's a vicious circle in this case. They are not hungry in the morning because they ate late the previous night. Since they don't eat in the morning, they tend to eat more towards the end of the day. If they eat more at once, blood sugar is unstable, which leaves them with cravings, especially at night. They can't lose weight for these obvious reasons, and we won't even touch the fact that they can't seem to sleep well enough. You clearly see that one bad habit could be feeding other ones. Let's reverse this. Let's start by cutting the bedtime snacks, which is no easy task but is the most rewarding one in my opinion. What will usually happen is that they start feeling hungry when they wake up. Since they now eat a little something first thing in the morning, the rest of the day doesn't seem to be as hard as it was before. More energy, no afternoon crash, controllable cravings and so on. Since the liver is at rest throughout the night, where it should be rejuvenating and producing growth hormones, the body starts regenerating and detoxifying efficiently again. Fat loss will most probably ensue.

Like Mary the lawyer, Niki the super-mom or Marty Brodeur, the elite NHL player, I had to figure out what could be the determining habit change that could kill two birds with one stone. However, my main goal with them and, I hope, with each and every one of you, is to show you what could happen when you change a few of these simple habits. How you feel, how it can change your days, how it can possibly impact your surroundings, your everyday life. Once you change that, it suddenly becomes harder to go back.

I truly hope from the bottom of my heart that the code will help you gain some control over your health. It's not as hard as we make ourselves believe. We just have to shut that voice in our head that makes us want to stay comfortable in that little routine that unintentionally made us take the wrong path. Be honest with yourself and recognize that little voice as soon as you hear it. Don't buy it. Our minds don't give a flying duck about what we want to achieve.

All they want is to stick with what we are doing, no change involved, sitting in its comfort zone. Our minds demand stability, but nothing gets done in the comfort of your own safety zone. Self-preservation is the main goal of all the cells in our body. They associate change with stress, but our cells don't actually differentiate between good and bad stress. Bad stress most often involves a prolonged period followed by physical or mental health issues, but good stress will be of short duration rewarded by the release of good, calming hormones and at times, an adrenaline rush, which makes our cells crave more. This is where it all begins. Once you find yourself stepping outside your safety zone, the feeling becomes addictive. You suddenly start craving a little more, still unsure if you want to jump completely out of the zone. Then, all you want is that feeling to come day in and day out. You want that feeling of tightness in the abdomen, the great workouts, the increased work performance, and more energy to go play with the kids at the park after a hard day's work. You want that feeling of being a lover to your wife or husband, not just being there to take out the garbage. You suddenly feel alive and loving every minute of it. I am not talking about going bungee jumping every day. All I want you to do is take control of your health and mind and to start living the rest of your life the way you deserve.

Your time is limited, so don't waste it living someone else's life. Don't be trapped by dogma - which is living with the results of other people's thinking. Don't let the noise of others' opinions drown out your own inner voice. And most importantly, have the courage to follow your heart and intuition.
— Steve Jobs

5530126R00085

Printed in Great Britain
by Amazon.co.uk, Ltd.,
Marston Gate.